LIVE WITH LOVE

Self Care Guide

Highlighting 52 *'ion'* Wellbeing Words

RAELENE DAL SANTO

Copyright © 2020 Raelene Dal Santo

Cover Design: Annie Seaton Author www.annieseaton.net

Cover Photo: Darius Bashar on Unsplash

Author Photo: Katrina Collins www.butterflymedia.marketing

Edited by: Mary Dal Santo and Annie Seaton

First Published 2020

Published by Raelene Dal Santo (Wellbeing Ways Australia)

PO Box 44 Macksville

NSW 2447 Australia

www.wellbeingways.com.au

All rights reserved. No part of this book may be reproduced by any mechanical, photographic, or electronic process, or in the form of a phonographic recording: nor may it be stored in a retrieval system, transmitted, or otherwise be copied for public or private use – other than 'fair use' as brief quotations embodied in articles and reviews – without the prior permission of the publisher. While every effort has been made to acknowledge the author of the quotes used, please contact the publisher if this has not occurred.

Disclaimer: The author of this book does not dispense medical advice or prescribe the use of any technique as a form of treatment for physical, emotional, or medical problems without the advice of a physician, either directly or indirectly. The intent of the author is only to offer information of a general nature to help you in your quest for emotional and spiritual wellbeing. In the event, you use any of the information in this book for yourself, the author and the publisher assume no responsibility for your actions.

Copyright © 2020 Raelene Dal Santo

All rights reserved.

ISBN-13: 978-0-6485410-0-4

DEDICATION

Thank you, Mum and Dad. You are my lifelong teachers and always demonstrate what it is to Live with Love.

Individually and together you give kindness and love and the world is a better place for these two precious gems you selflessly share.

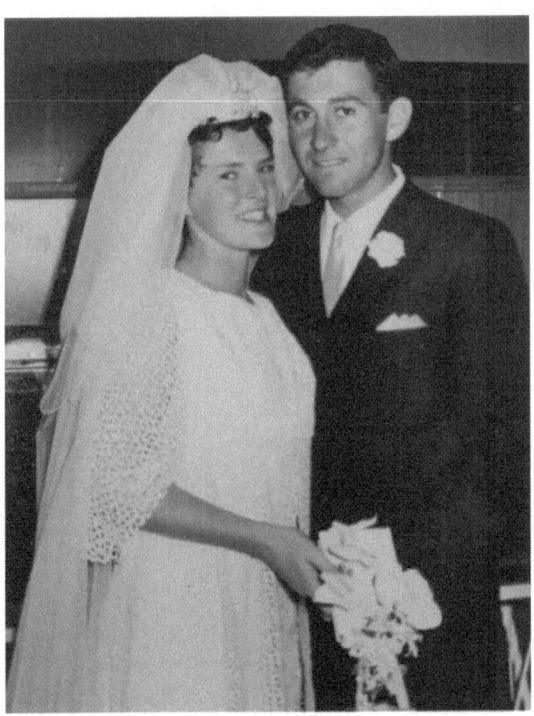

RAELENE DAL SANTO

CONTENTS

Introduction

1. **Live with Love** — 7
2. ***'ion'* Your Life** — 12
3. **How to use this book.** — 19
4. **Lifestyle Wellbeing Ways to *'ion'* your life** — 25

   (See Index p212 for *'ion'* page numbers)
5. **Life is Love. Love is Life.** — 205
6. **References and Suggested Readings** — 208

   Index — 212

ACKNOWLEDGMENTS

♥ Mum: You have a heart full of love, a soul full of kindness and fun, and a mind full of wisdom and knowledge. You always believe in me. You encourage and remind me to share a smile, sprinkle magic and live with kindness as love made visible. Thank you for being my Angel, guiding Lighthouse, Literary Superstar, cheer squad and life coach. I love you two bob.

♥ Dad: Family and kindness are at the heart of your being. You like everything kind and calm, and these are two magical ingredients the world deserves. Thank you for your support and love. You are my superhero. I love you.

♥ To my brothers Peter, David and Anthony; sister in laws Trish, Emma and Jo; nieces Kyrah, Mikayla, Aleah, Darcy and Jessica; nephews Jake, Keaton, Jackson and Brendan and their families; aunts, uncles, cousins and all my family and friends, I am who I am because of your contribution to my life. A little bit of everything I have learned from each of you is in this book. Thank you for your time, kindness, generosity of heart and love.

♥ Thank you to Nanna, Grandad Jack, Grandma and Grandad Don guiding from above.

♥ Thank you to the students, staff and communities I have had the privilege to be a part of.

♥ Annie Seaton Author: Thank you for the cover design,

editing expertise and for sharing your publishing knowledge and wisdom.

♥Jane Dans: Thank you for your friendship, support and encouragement. Three valued and treasured gifts.

♥Fiona McArthur Author: Thank you for the gift of 'commit to writing five hundred words a day' as your wise words are now this book.

♥Maureen Noonan: Thank you Aunty M for your encouragement, inspiration, literary guidance and publishing wisdom.

♥Michelle Welsh: Thank you for your friendship, support and listening ear as I talked through ideas.

♥Sue Larkey: Thank you for being my soul sister and for always believing in me. Your kindness and wisdom help children, families and communities all over the world.

♥Sue E. Larkey: Thank you for your support, love and encouragement to follow my dreams.

♥Tamara Mc William: Thank you for your friendship, being a technical guru, sharing your time, publishing insights and business experience. May your books fly with wings all over the world.

LIVE WITH LOVE

Self Care Guide

Highlighting 52 *'ion'* Wellbeing Words

The secret of getting ahead is getting started. - Mark Twain

The essence of this book is for 'younique' you.

Love your life. Create your life. Enjoy your life.

Remember to *Live with Love*.

Let's begin your self care Wellbeing Ways journey with the magic of fifty-two *'ion'* words and hundreds of practical activities.

Love Raelene

RAELENE DAL SANTO

INTRODUCTION

It is nine days' post operation and I am home alone. I can't drive. I can't move. I can't think.

The following diary excerpt is what inspired me to write this book to help you create and live a life of wellness, kindness, calmness, happiness and success.

'You survived the big C' and 'You may not have been here to see forty-eight,' are the words. In a moment, they simultaneously took my breath away, and made me grateful for the breath of life.

Puzzled, I asked, "Did you call the right patient?"

Stunned and shocked, I nervously giggled and repeatedly thought, 'I'm okay. I'm okay. I'm okay.' I reminded myself, 'I will make it to forty-eight, I am living to 103.'

As I called loved ones, I remembered three things from the call. We got it all. It was occult. Your job is to heal.

I thought to myself; it is time to heal, to reset, to let go, to change, to love, to write.

This book is for you. A self care guide for you to turn the page, tick your bucket list, live your dreams and 'make someday, one day, today.'

Create self care changes so you can connect and thrive, living and enjoying a life you love.

1. LIVE WITH LOVE

Love as an overriding principle

If love is an overriding principle, then it is above personal quests. The principle of love challenges, hurts and causes reflection at the core of ourselves and of society. The aim of this book is to cross all barriers so that all humanity, across all cultures and all countries can shine and *Live with Love*. Love will look different for everyone, as does your life, lifestyle and expression of love.

If you love your life, your chosen work, career, study or lifestyle, then that is truly great. It is a gift. This book is to inspire you to further develop to *Live with Love* and explore your connectedness and relationships with your family, friends, partner and yourself. It extends to hobbies and interests, finances, health and wellbeing, spirituality, career, study or work. It is important to foster the connectedness of yourself with all aspects of your life. This takes time, attention and action. So, if you are happy with one aspect of your life, this book is designed to look at opportunities that you may not have thought of or even know about.

You, I, and everyone goes about living their life, and like the lyrics from *Beautiful Boy* by John Lennon, 'Life is what happens to you while you're busy making other plans.'

Each day, life gives us both expected and unexpected things to deal with whether these be situations or people. You get to choose in each situation how you act. Everyone is at different ages and stages of life. Everyone has a 'younique' experience of interpreting the world. Everyone else is not the 'younique' individual you are.

As you read, try any activity that speaks to you. This book is designed to be practical and fun, to guide you to discover ways to live your purpose and passion, create your intention and direction and create actions to *Live with Love*.

Thrive vs Survive

Everybody lives a different life. My wise Mum says, 'You never know what happens behind someone's eyes.' This means, no one knows what it is like to be you and you don't know what it is like to be someone else. Stop living up to someone else's expectation and stop expecting someone else to live up to yours. Compassion, empathy and understanding sprinkled with large quantities of the magic of kindness and love, are key ingredients to being with someone that understands you and you them.

This life, your life, is traversed with mountains, rivers and oceans both geographically and personal. It may be that things seem to be as big and as overwhelming as these large natural gifts. Sometimes what you are dealing with appears large. It can become all-consuming and negative. Overwhelming thoughts can consume and distract you from the positive in life. You may be bombarded by one thing after another, after another. This happens. It could take you to the 'why me', 'what is happening', and the 'I need help' moments. This is where the gift of love comes in. This includes self-love and love for and from others.

There are always moments in life to choose how you respond to a certain situation. Life constantly presents change in people, places, things and situations for you to assess and choose what action to take. As the Greek philosopher Heraclitus says, 'Change is the only constant in life.' Humans are like a wave. A wave is a disturbance moving through a medium. Your thoughts and physical body are constantly changing through the journey of life.

Times of your focus vs focus of your time

At certain times in life, you can be focused on your goals and intentions. At other times, things seem to be given precedence and happenings triaged, according to circumstance. That is life. We all have times of focus and at other times, things have our focus. Too often we make ourselves wrong for not starting or completing something.

What stops some people and why do others proceed? Everyone is different, so different. The most important relationship in your life is the one you have with yourself. Your energy changes each day. Life is a series of days, each with a beginning and an end. Life has structure and yet is unstructured for you to create your world.

Fear holds us back and love moves us forward. Fear can be a duality; in that you could be afraid of success or failure. Either can be a grip like effect. Like traffic lights, you could feel stopped at a red light or unable to make choices to keep going or to stop, like the orange light.

What makes the light of the green light shine, is what you may be searching for. How can today be a little better than yesterday? How can you find that little spark that would make all the difference? How can you let your light shine?

At times, everyone holds themselves back for whatever the reason. By putting yourself in situations that take you out of your comfort zone, you may achieve results and have unexpected, exciting outcomes. This book gives you the opportunity to explore what you would like for you.

Positive Psychology

Positive psychology has many definitions, related meanings, concepts, frameworks and opinions. My interpretation of this term is the scientific study of humans and applied applications of thriving functioning individuals, organisations and communities: be it local, national or global.

With that, my aim is to share ideas, thoughts, experiences,

words and practical strategies for you to apply to your life. Use these to create a spark, remind you to be grateful, help you discover your purpose and passion, and to thrive vs survive.

This book combines my life experiences, skills, and knowledge as a registered teacher for more than thirty years, registered integrated massage therapist, studies in journalism and hospitality - patisserie.

You will discover hundreds of practical ideas to choose from, and then apply, so you can be a thriving functioning individual. You will notice this book is about choice. It is designed to be progressive rather than prescriptive. Since everyone's reason for change and access to resources, both personal and physical vary, choose what appeals to you and your lifestyle.

2. *'ION'* YOUR LIFE

Thrive vs Survive
A positive attitude from you tends to produce a positive attitude toward you.
- Deborah Day

Wherever I went, I heard or saw *'ion'* words. To me, they symbolise action and are inspiring and empathic.

An *ion* is an atom, or molecule, with a total electric charge a result of a gain or loss of one or more electrons. Apologies to any physicists, but in simple terms, that is, the total number of electrons is not equal to the total number of protons, this giving the atom, or the molecule a net positive or negative electrical charge. Stay with me, so an *ion,* has a positive or negative charge.

This book shares, learning about, learning from, and letting go anything negative that does not serve you anymore whilst also creating space, and letting in something positive that now serves your life.

Life is a constant flow of energy. Deborah Day, author of *Be Happy Now: Become the Active Director of your Life,* said 'Positive energy is attracted to positive energy.' Energy is a constant. It is always around but flow and its rhythms can change.

How do you know if it is time to release or gain? Only you will know. Your life story is different from anyone else's. Your background, experiences, knowledge, skills and interactions differ from another's. You see things from different angles. You experience life through filters of your senses differently. No matter how I word this, life is different for you than for anyone not you. You truly are an individual.

Using the *'ion'* words

You can use the *'ion'* words in any combination you like, there are no rules. The words are a stimulus for you to use, to activate, create and look at any part of your life you choose to address, change or admire.

Like art, nothing is wrong, it is an interpretation from perspective, both that of the artist and that of the viewer. Like life, it is all a matter of perspective, from filters and from experiences. Respect and honour where you are at. Respect and honour where someone else is at. Honour your journey. Honour their journey.

Self-love, self-nurture and self-expression are not selfish, they are selfless. No one knows you like you do, and if you do not take care of you, who can, and who will? Plan, create and *'ion'* your life, and *Live with Love.*

Maslow's Hierarchy of Needs

Psychologist Abraham Maslow's hierarchy of needs is a developmental psychology theory of the patterns of human motivation. His paper *A Theory of Human Motivation* appeared in *Psychology Review,* in 1943. I was introduced to this theory at university in 1990 and it continues to fascinate me. Maslow refined his theory over decades: 1942, 1962 and 1987. In his theory, Maslow used the words *physiological, safety, belonging/love, esteem, self-actualisation* and *self-transcendence.*

His theory is about human behaviour motivated by attaining these needs. An individual may not necessarily move through the hierarchy pyramid in a vertical direction. Rather, depending on circumstances, may move between the different needs at differing times. Maslow was interested in how humans fulfil human potential. You will notice with the fifty-two *'ion'* words used in this book, I refer to many of the activities of human being, rather than doing or having.

For this book and my message, I have used *'ion'* words to share years of study and experience. To illustrate Maslow's theory, I have used as a comparison the following *'ion'* words to demonstrate the physiological and other parts of Maslow's theory from the hierarchical pyramid.

To gain further understanding of these *'ion'* words used, refer to the index. Each is defined and outlined in more detail with practical ways to wellbeing in Chapter 4. If you are interested, you may like to read further about Maslow's theories in his book *Motivation and Personality,* and other publications since its release in 1954.

If you choose to research Maslow, you will soon discover there are various drawings of the hierarchical needs pyramid. For the purposes of this book, I have correlated my *'ion'* words with Maslow's words, from the base word *physiological,* then *safety, love/belonging, esteem* and *self-actualisation,* at the top of the pyramid.

Physiological needs
Hydrat*ion* - water
Nutrit*ion* - food
Ventilat*ion* - breathing and clean air
Accommodat*ion* - shelter
Fash*ion* – clothing or covering for protection or social context
Mot*ion* - activity and exercise

Safety needs
Protect*ion* - of self and others
Vocat*ion* - study and work
Pass*ion* - purpose or focus

Love/Belonging needs
Affect*ion* - for self, others and life
Affiliat*ion* - to groups and organisations
Connect*ion* - to self and others

Esteem needs
Appreciat*ion* - of self and others

Self-actualisation needs
Cognit*ion* - knowledge acquisition and understanding
Beautificat*ion* - appealing to the senses
Creat*ion* - creativity
Compass*ion* - of self and others
Opin*ion* - acceptance

Self-realisa*tion* - life lessons
Self-regual*tion* - monitor, maintain and alter behaviour

52 *'ion'* words

Every day your energy changes and who you are today is different from yesterday and will be different from tomorrow. A new day represents an opportunity for a new beginning.

The following is a list of *'ion'* words chosen for this book. Obviously, there are many others, but these fulfilled the need for my research and for what I want to share, so you can live your dreams. You will discover hundreds of practical self care ideas for you to transform your wellbeing, connect with what matters and thrive in your world.

Read the following list and choose words that interest or appeal to you.

1. Accommodation
2. Action
3. Affection
4. Affiliation
5. Appreciation
6. Beautification
7. Celebration
8. Cognition
9. Collection
10. Communication
11. Companion
12. Compassion
13. Congratulation

14. Connection
15. Consumption
16. Cooperation
17. Creation
18. Detoxification
19. Direction
20. Education
21. Energisation
22. Expression
23. Fashion
24. Generation
25. Hydration
26. Impression
27. Information
28. Innovation
29. Inspiration
30. Location
31. Meditation
32. Motion
33. Motivation
34. Nutrition
35. Observation
36. Opinion
37. Organisation
38. Passion
39. Preparation
40. Protection
41. Reflection
42. Rejuvenation
43. Relaxation
44. Satisfaction

45. Self-realisation
46. Self-regulation
47. Sensation
48. Tradition
49. Transformation
50. Vacation
51. Ventilation
52. Vocation

3. HOW TO USE THIS BOOK

Thrive vs Survive

This chapter is the magic of the book, my favourite part, the ingredients for the recipe to create something for yourself. It is for you to discover your direction and passion, and move from intention to action, and *Live with Love*.

Try an *'ion'* practical idea daily, or weekly. Connect with family and friends and if you create your own *'ion'* self care activities, I encourage you to share and email me or use #52ionwellbeingways. Remember that change in your life happens from releasing or changing something that does not serve you anymore. Try something new or something that you may have known about but needed a reminder to implement in your life. Now. Today.

What does each *'ion'* word offer you?

Each *'ion'* word has/a:

- Five lifestyle Wellbeing Ways
- Quotation
- Notation
- Thrive on five
- *'ion'* word summary

Each one is explained as follows:

Five Lifestyle Wellbeing Ways to *'ion'* your life

A suggestion of lifestyle ways to use the ideas written for each *'ion'* word.

Quotation

Each word commences with an inspiring quote. Words linger long after they are spoken or written in your thoughts. Words can impact you on a soul level, inspiring you, guiding you, and teaching you. Words are what distinguishes humans from other animals. Words can linger in thoughts for many moments, so this book is about the positive and kind words and deeds for yourself and others.

Notation

The notation section is information and inspiration, a blurb or summation on the fifty-two *'ion'* words. It represents thoughts, explanations and ideas to empower you to use this word and choose where it will fit into your lifestyle. You may have different interpretations or translations, that's okay, use it how it works for you.

Thrive on Five

This section contains the practical strategies devised as a guide to add the magic of the *'ion'* words into your life. The fifty-two *'ion'* words have practical ideas for you to choose ways of being for wellness, happiness, kindness, calmness and success.

Word Summary

This is five key points about each *'ion' word*. The words are in alphabetical order for ease of finding them. Remember, this book is about choice. It is progressive not prescriptive. Try something familiar or try something new. Love. Create. Enjoy.

52 Lifestyle Wellbeing Ways to *'ion'* your life

This is my favourite part. These are fifty-two *'ion'* words and practical self care wellbeing ways to live your dreams and a life you love.

Read the following list with the '5 Lifestyle Wellbeing Ways' heading section. Again, if a word or an activity resonates then note it, so you can come back later and discover how you can incorporate the idea to suit your lifestyle.

1. Accommodation: five thoughts on being home or away
2. Action: five ways to move from intention to action
3. Affection: five ideas to make moments count with love
4. Affiliation: five nurturing ways to create belonging
5. Appreciation: five thoughtful ways of being thankful
6. Beautification: five glimpses of human nature and Mother Nature
7. Celebration: five heartfelt ways to share joy
8. Cognition: five thoughtful ways to use your master-

mind
9. Collection: five views on trash or treasure
10. Communication: five ways to share your true essence
11. Companion: five thoughtful ways to nourish your soul
12. Compassion: five nurturing viewpoints of self and others
13. Congratulation: five ways to express success and happiness
14. Connection: five relationship views of self, others and the universe
15. Consumption: five observances of human connectedness
16. Cooperation: five unifying reminders of human difference yet sameness
17. Creation: five ways to discover creativity within and around you
18. Detoxification: five nurturing ways to release what no longer serves you
19. Direction: five thoughts on choosing what matters to you
20. Education: five benefits of teaching and learning
21. Energisation: five recharging ways to energise your life
22. Expression: five ways to discover your 'love made visible' to the world
23. Fashion: five ways to express your individuality
24. Generation: five respectful ways of generational teaching and learning
25. Hydration: five thoughts on why water is liquid gold
26. Impression: five thoughtful ways of interacting
27. Information: five views on knowledge and human

connectedness
28. Innovation: five approaches to create with courage
29. Inspiration: five ideas for positive practice
30. Location: five ideas to be right here and right now
31. Meditation: five nurturing and restorative ways of being
32. Motion: five ways to create a vision and venture to achieve it
33. Motivation: five inspiring ways to action your goals and dreams
34. Nutrition: five ways food sustains life
35. Observation: five ways to notice the beauty of life
36. Opinion: five ways to embrace life with grace
37. Organisation: five compassionate ways to make a difference
38. Passion: five ways to discover and live your dreams
39. Preparation: five ways to conceive, believe and achieve success
40. Protection: five ways of providing a sanctuary for self, others, nature and ideas
41. Reflection: five ways life mirrors a message to you
42. Rejuvenation: five guiding ways to regenerate your spirit
43. Relaxation: five gems to create 'soulitude'
44. Satisfaction: five nourishing ways to achieve what you need and want
45. Self-realisation: five reminders of learning life lessons in every moment
46. Self-regulation: five ways to monitor, maintain or alter your behaviour in each moment
47. Sensation: five ways to allow yourself to feel it to heal

it
48. Tradition: five guiding ideas on the sameness and newness of habits and customs
49. Transformation: five reminders of the journey not the destination of life
50. Vacation: five ideas to homestay or getaway
51. Ventilation: five observances for every breath you take
52. Vocation: five lifestyle ideas for your study, job or career

4. LIFESTYLE WELLBEING WAYS TO *'ION'* YOUR LIFE

52 *'ion'* words and practical self care wellbeing ways to live your dreams and a life you love.

5 thoughts on being home or away

1. Accommodat*ion*

Quotation
Wherever I lay my hat (That's my home) – Song by Marvin Gaye, Barrett Strong and Norman Whitfield

Notation
Accommodation varies depending upon your lifestyle and circumstances, but generally it is a place in which you live, work, learn, or stay and most facets of lifestyle come under these three areas. It could be temporary or permanent.

Accommodation is planned and built according to the availability of raw materials, the environment, any legislative requirements and the specific needs for whom and where it is intended. It is designed to meet the needs of a populous or a potential population and again, it can be temporary or permanent. Changing accommodation by moving home, decluttering, visiting, travelling, or rearranging furniture and décor, helps you thrive as this phrase suggests, 'a change is as good as a holiday.'

Thrive on Five

1. Reduce. Reuse. Recycle
What could you do to reduce the single use items in your home? What could you reuse and create a multifunction for? What could you recycle instead of sending to landfill? What household items could you rearrange? Decluttering allows for physical clearing and the emotional attachment to it. Shedding allows you to feel lighter and the energy to change within and around you. What could you release?

2. Dream Home
Do you dream of finding a home that caters for your needs and wants? Do you draw or sketch designs? Do you take photos of structures you like? Do you research buildings already constructed with similar needs? Is there anyone you know who could artistically and skilfully create your dream home? Your home is your castle. It is not to be compared to anyone else's, because if it serves your needs and fulfils your wants, then it is a home. Your home. If you own your dream home, but need a change, you could redecorate by arranging items or create statement pieces.

3. The Universe is your home
With the world population being ever transient and the access to travel ever available, home is the universe. Travellers are out and about taking their home on the road, seeing places, meeting people and experiencing life. Travelling is for any age and stage of your life. Your needs and wants will determine the destination. Have fun on the journey. Travel with direction or laidback intention. Create and enjoy experiences.

4. Homelessness

Sometimes people have no home, some have accommodation to go to but choose not to or can't go there. This is a global issue, what could you do to help at a local level? Who or what organisation could you offer help or resources to? What could you reduce, reuse or recycle so that someone else may use and benefit from?

5. Holiday havens

If you are wanting or needing a holiday, you could have guests in your home, house swap or house sit. Be creative. There are websites for all these options, both nationally and internationally. Of course, with any of these suggestions you need to use your judgement and check specific details both legislative and protective.

Accommodat*ion* Summary

- Everyone's lifestyle is different.
- Lifestyle for some is a choice, others are not afforded such freedom.
- Be where you want to live with whom you want to live with.
- The universe population is increasingly transient and accessible.
- Accommodation varies depending on the needs and wants of the population.

LIVE WITH LOVE

5 ways to move from intention to action

2. Act*ion*

Quotation

Do you want to know who you are? Don't ask. Act! Action will delineate and define you. – Thomas Jefferson

Notation

Benjamin Franklin said, 'Well done is better than well said.' Fear stops you acting but action takes courage and helps build confidence. If you do not take actions no matter how small, in the direction of your dreams, they remain that. Someone dear to me said, 'Do what is in front of you, one step at a time.' This will lead you to the next action and the next one. It is like sport. Some watch. Some play. Some coach. Some dream. Which one are you? Do you turn to abstraction instead of action? Do you feel stuck at the orange traffic light of life, or worse the red? Are you gathering information, rather than applying it? Do you sit on the side, hoping one day, someday but take no action to achieve it? Do you coach and lift others by your guidance to be the best they can be? Do you play the game of life and know that sometimes you will win, sometimes you take risks, but always, you learn about yourself and others?

Thrive on Five

1. Start acting vs wishful thinking

How often have you felt like you are at the orange traffic light of life? Or even the red? The inaction grips you as fear takes an acute hold. It prevents you from action as you feel protected by the slow inaction. Not choosing is a choice but you forget that in the pain. Action, taking opportunities and learning lessons is the key. What action could you take to move one step closer to your dream? Who could you ask for help? Be in action instead of wishful thinking into the future. Turn someday, one day, into today.

2. Action vs procrastination

Planning is to produce action. Stagnation of an idea or concept is procrastination. Your perspective is the way you see something. If you look at it from a different spot, or from someone else's perspective you may realise possibilities that you did not even know existed. Mum reminds me, 'So called failure is one step closer to success.' As a young teacher with three years' experience it was difficult to get a position when I moved to a new state within Australia. I couldn't get a job in the public system unless I had a number to teach, but as it was, you couldn't get a number to teach unless you had a job. So, I applied for any educational positions and commenced as a teacher's aide. This led to teaching positions, leadership roles and all add up to the experience of today. Create long term and short term goals and small steps to mastery towards your dream. Take one action today. Who will you be? Courageous? Outrageous? Confident? Brave? You choose your action and who you will be in that moment.

3. Step forward vs continual planning

Step forward and be in action. Sometimes this is scary and overwhelming and the 'what ifs' could take over. Planning is necessary for success but without action it remains a plan, a dream, a someday, one day. For the writing of this book I have spoken with successful people in their chosen field and they all say that they started somewhere. Where it led them to today is the wonderful web that connects humanity. We are all connected. So, life is therefore a collection of connections. We are all on our own journey of life. What could you plan, then take one step at a time to make it happen? What action could you take today toward your dream? Call someone. Send an email. Ask a question. Teach a skill. Research. Move from the creativity with the mind to the action of the body.

4. Start playing vs just observing

Stop observing someone else's life and live your own. Often in this transient and digital world it is all too easy to see others achieve their dream. Stop comparing. Stop observing. Start playing. Start living. Remember, a sporting team trains and plans for the game, but only by playing do they find out if they are victorious or not. Both victory and defeat give lessons to tweak for even better performances. Playing is action. Not playing is wishful thinking. Where in life could you stop observing and start playing the game of life?

5. Teaching and Learning

We are all teachers and learners. A degree gives a qualification, but you do not need one to teach someone something. You need to be open to learning and possibilities, and willing to teach and share with others. I learned from many teachers about the process of publishing this book. Learning is the essential ingredient for progress. Learning must happen in your world and around you, not in abstract. Planning is to produce action, not for the stagnation of an idea or concept. This is procrastination.

Act*ion* Summary

- Are you a dreamer, an observer, a coach, a player or a combination?
- Take an action that leads you towards your dream.
- Seek out those that can help you achieve your dream.
- Everyone starts somewhere.
- *Live with Love*. Be in action.

5 ideas to make moments count with love

3. Affect*ion*

Quotation
Affection is the feeling of liking or endearment or love of somewhere, something or someone. This is also self care and devotion for others. – Raelene Dal Santo

Notation
Self-nourishment, self care, self-love and self-respect are all acts of being selfless, not selfish. The most important relationship you will have is the one with yourself. Nurture yourself. If you find this hard to read, difficult to envisage, unable to know where to find the time, money or resources then be creative. Make time. Manage time. Ask for assistance. Be social. Connect with family and friends. Take your lunch break. Wake up early. Be creative. Eat well. Sleep. Exercise. Hydrate. Relax. Decrease stress. Speak your truth. Be kind to yourself. Write and unload your thoughts onto paper. Be expressive and be open to learn ways to support your physical, emotional, social, mental, and spiritual wellbeing.

Thrive on Five

1. Develop your nurture network

Develop your own nurture network of trustworthy family, friends and colleagues you can turn to for support. Relationships can teach us about ourselves and allow us to contribute to the lives of others. Nurture networks can assist you to be responsible, respectful and resilient in good times and nurture you when support is needed. This increases your sense of belonging.

2. Gratitude

Be thankful for those who contribute to your life and let them know you appreciate their kindness and generosity. Someone's time and energy are gifts, contributing to your life. Accept their help and allow their contribution. Remember, relationships are two way, so be available to listen, support and help others when needed. Be respectful of your own needs. Be respectful of others' needs. Sometimes this requires balance.

3. Detox. Shetox. Hetox.

Whatever this is for you, remove unwanted energy for yourself. This could be people, places, or things. Seek assistance from family, friends, energy healers or health care professionals to assist you to do this. Clean out. Dispose. Donate. Remove from your life what no longer serves you. Declutter to flutter and shine.

4. Volunteer

Sometimes directing energy to assist others, helps you. It does not solve any matter you may be dealing with, but it will give you a different perspective. Be generous with your time. Giving is receiving. This applies to yourself as well as to others. Give without expectation. Receive with gratitude. Where could you volunteer your resources of time and energy?

5. Pets as Therapy

The spontaneity of animals, being in the here and now, needing the provision of food and shelter for survival, can also give affection for the provider. Pets as therapy organisations offer therapeutic visits to schools, hospitals, homes and care facilities. This can play an important role in enhancing social, emotional, physical and mental wellbeing. Could you or someone you know, benefit from a pet to enhance wellbeing?

Affect*ion* Summary

- What are your passions?
- Who in your life is your nurture network?
- What activities, ideas, tools and techniques do you use to make you a well-being?
- What do you need to release from your life?
- What volunteer organisation could use your talents, time and energy?

5 nurturing ways to create belonging

4. Affiliat*ion*

Quotation

Everyone can be a leader irrespective of their age, race, creed, nationality or political affiliation. Once you figure out your talents and optimise them very well, at the right place and at the right time, you are a leader. – Israelmore Aylvor

Notation

Do you belong to any organisations or groups? Do you have an affiliation with a community group, person, place or thing? Being part of a group allows for the sharing of common interests, skills and experiences. It also allows for connections or meeting with others on a local, national and international basis, or via the world of digital connection. Learning a new skill is cognitively beneficial and connectedness with others allows for mental, emotional, physical and social wellbeing. Research groups in your area that interest you. Could you start a group?

Thrive on Five

1. Find, or create your affiliation

Whether you are interested in an outdoor or indoor pursuit, there is an organisation, group, affiliation, or committee for you to join. If not, then create it. Rosemary Shiparo-Lou author of *The Mentor Within,* created Global Walking Tribe. It is a tribe that walks for thirty minutes per day, wherever you are, whenever you like. How fabulous.

2. Affiliate yourself

The following list is not conclusive, just for consideration. Sew. Draw. Paint. Sculpt. Weave. Quilt. Bake. Cook. Decorate. Garden. Farm. Write. Read. Direct. Design. Clean. Photograph. Build. Manage. Run. Walk. Surf. Paddle. Fly. Swim. Cycle. Bush walk. Plant. Collect. Climb. Jump. Organise. Sail. Fix. Construct. Speak. Listen. Sport. Music. Sing. Dance. Play. Study. Learn. Teach. Care. Protect. Help. What have you chosen?

3. Helping Others

Who do you know, or what organisation could you help to foster social, emotional, mental or physical wellbeing and connectedness for others? Sometimes when your focus is not you, but others, the gift of kindness benefits everyone. Dr David R Hamilton shares this message in his book, *The Five Side Effects of Kindness.* Kindness in its true essence, is a gift from the heart, and the world could always do with heart-fullness. Quietly do a kind act.

4. Nature and conservation organisations

There are many local, national or global organisations that could use your skills, knowledge, experience and enthusiasm. Here are a few to consider: Local or native endangered animals or abandoned animals, international organisations for the conservation of native land and the protection of animals, the protection of farmlands and waterways, causes for children or elderly, and those for the protection of human rights. Do you have a qualification, skill or experience that could benefit an affiliation or cause? Could you contribute your valuable time and energy, either in a paid or voluntary role?

5. Your vibe and tribe

Life is about every moment, acknowledging the past, looking to the future and remembering to live in the now. These are more than clichéd words. Calmness and peace may be finding your passion, living with passion, finding time to nurture your soul, being with people that 'get you,' and in turn allow you to contribute to their life. Being with a tribe with a similar vibe lifts you up, enlivens your soul and supports you to be who you would like to be. The tribe could be family, friends, colleagues, teachers, students, or community organisations.

Affiliat*ion* Summary

- Where in your life are you a leader?
- What group or organisation would you like to belong to? Join in.
- Use your gifts and talents, don't let them go unnoticed or unused.
- How could you help others with your 'youniqueness?'
- Take care of nature and allow Mother Nature to take care of you.

5 thoughtful ways of being thankful

5. Appreciat*ion*

Quotation
When you are grateful, fear disappears, and abundance appears. – Tony Robbins

Notation
The teachings of the late Louise Hay made me more conscious of the words I think and speak and how I listen to others. I read her book, *The Power is Within You*, as a young adult and discovered the use of affirmations as positive words to affirm in present tense, as if what you were saying or thinking, already existed in the here and now.

Whilst studying for my degree a couple of years earlier, I was fortunate to study the teachings in the book *People Skills*, by Robert Bolton. As the book says, it is about, 'How to assert yourself, listen to others, and resolve conflicts.' It is as essential today for effective communication skills and appreciating your own and others perspective, as it was when first published, in 1979.

Thrive on Five

1. Having an attitude of gratitude

Write in a gratitude journal daily being grateful for everything in your life. Be sure to note the little things that you may take for granted. Watch for the daily acts of kindness bestowed to you. Be conscious of receiving a smile, a hug, a thank you and tasks or requests completed. Be grateful for food to eat, clean water to drink, a bed to sleep in, a home, family, friends, money, a job or business. Notice. Notice. Notice and be grateful.

2. Thank you

Two simple words. Heartfelt, heart-given, heart received. Notice random and intended acts of kindness. Observe. Write thank you cards, emails, notes and make calls. Acknowledge and be grateful for a kind deed. Valuing and respecting the generosity of someone or something they did, shows recognition of your enjoyment and your appreciation. Your gratitude will be welcomed. Giving is from the heart without the expectation of receiving. The words thank you, are too often unsaid and unheard but much valued. Notice when someone does something for you or of themselves. Whether a child, parent, sibling, colleague, peer, friend, family member, store attendant, stranger, or even someone you pay to complete a transaction or service, remember the common courtesy of thank you. Kindness begets kindness. Dr David R Hamilton author of *The Five Side Effects of Kindness,* shares that these are: 'It makes us happier, is good for the heart, slows ageing, improves relationships and is contagious.'

3. Family just as it is

The people that constitute a family, varies in each home,

community or country. Family are our first teachers. They guide us from dependence to independence and their teachings expose us to the interdependence of all humans. Family are our lifelong teachers. As an educator for more than thirty years I have heard, 'They will teach that at school.' Many curricular, extracurricular, social, emotional, and physical skills are taught at school, but consider the symbiotic relationship of working together works best. Teachers may have an impact for a certain time, but again, parents or caregivers are lifelong teachers. Never underestimate the importance of family, whatever that looks like in your life. In family, we learn survival strategies. It is love that extends this.

4. The role of significant others

The impact of childhood and adolescence is lifelong. When I listened to my grandparents, aunts and uncles share stories or recounts of their life, it was mostly about these years. I enjoy listening to family and friends. I like to listen to why people do what they do? My brother wisely said to me, 'If you listen and learn one thing from each person you meet, you will learn a lot of wisdom.'

5. Pay it forward

Pay it Forward is a novel by Catherine Ryan Hyde. This book has a simple message, in that starting with your own world, you can change the world. A teacher with a vision gave his class an assignment and a boy, together with his altruism, an idea and time, changed his world, and the world. The lyrics of the song, *From Little Things, Big Things Grow*, by Paul Kelly and Kev Carmody are very apt here. It is a reminder to just start somewhere and work towards your goal. The ripple effect is never-ending, and you may never see or know the effects of your efforts and kindness, but the world will. Kindness is a good place to start.

Appreciat*ion* Summary

- Appreciate what you have whilst you have it.
- Being grateful benefits the giver as well as the receiver.
- Give with all your heart without expectation of receiving.
- Share the ripple effect of kindness as it is love made visible.
- Gratitude allows you to notice and appreciate abundance.

5 glimpses of human nature and Mother Nature

6. Beautific*ion*

Quotation
Beauty is in the eyes of the beholder. – Proverb

Notation
This quote is like all areas of life, in that what one person likes or may find beautiful, may not appeal to another. Everyone is different, our likes and dislikes of people, places and things. That is okay, and with understanding, we must all be respectful.

Thrive on Five

1. Notice the beauty within and around you
Often you may do things without noticing things and people around you. Today, look up and look around and take time to stop and observe. Notice everything around you. The home you live in, the people in your world, the architecture, the cars, the transport, or nature. Notice and observe. Beauty exists within and around you all the time. Take time to notice.

2. The beauty of nature
Nature is a reminder of all the wondrous natural gifts that exist in the world. This includes but is not exclusive to birds, animals, flora, wildlife, oceans, rivers, lakes, creeks, mountains, farmlands, sunrise, sunset and people. Nature can teach you many life lessons. Notice. Observe. Appreciate.

3. The beauty in people
People exist across the world and are the collective of human beings. Members of families, communities and countries may vary outwardly, but collectively share beauty within. Notice acts of kindness throughout your day. Share some kindness today with those in your world. The free smile you give today, may be a welcome gift for someone else to receive. Share beauty in the world. Notice the qualities of others. Value difference.

4. Project or cause
What activity, whether paid or unpaid deserves your time and attention. Is there a cause close to your heart that you could give your time and energy, that would make a difference to an individual, group or the world? Choose it and add your 'younique' gifts to enhance this cause for yourself, or for others.

Projects bring people together for a common cause.

5. Beauty within

Be present to yourself and your 'youniqueness'. Take time to discover what beautification means to you. Beautification is something that appeals to your senses. You can add beauty to the world by being 'younique' you and sharing your talents, skills, ideas and heart.

Beautification Summary

- You add beauty to the world.
- Beauty is within.
- Mother Nature's beauty is ever present.
- Look for the beauty within others.
- Share your 'younique' talents with a cause or project.

5 heartfelt ways to share joy

7. Celebration

Quotation

Every day is a good day. There is always something to learn, celebrate and be grateful for. – Mary Dal Santo

Notation

The joy of being alive is a gift. Rajneesh (born Chandra Moran Jain) said, 'Celebration is my attitude, unconditional to what life brings.' Whatever is going on in your life celebrate each moment, express gratitude and appreciation. Each day gives opportunities to offer gratitude or congratulations to people and wish them well for their wellness, happiness and success.

Thrive on Five
1. Lessons learned
Oprah Winfrey said, 'The more you praise and celebrate your life, the more there is in life to celebrate.' Celebrate the successes you achieve and be grateful for the so-called failures and celebrate the new lessons learned. How do you celebrate your success? How do you acknowledge your life lessons? Both perceived victories and defeats are your teachers and you the student of the lesson. Every situation has a learning opportunity.

2. Celebration party
What or who could you celebrate? Organise a cultural, religious, thank you, engagement, graduation, birthday, anniversary, neighbourhood, family, friend, work, study, or community celebration. The main part of this is the acknowledgement, of the contribution of others to something, some cause or someone.

3. Award or reward others
Who could you nominate for an award in recognition for their contribution to community or for an area of humanity? Think local, national or global recognition. Look around you, in your world, not just in the media or the digital world. Who are the quiet achievers, the silent contributors, everyday philanthropists, the carers of the world, or the volunteers of the world? Who are the ones who give generously from their heart in the true sense of giving that you could recognise?

4. Celebrate today
Be present to the gift that you are. Each day is a new beginning.

It is an opportunity for renewal. Celebrate who you are in your heart and who you know yourself to be to others. Love yourself. Be kind to yourself. Forgive yourself. Life is a journey and continual lessons appear on the path. Today is the day you could choose to change something in your life. If you choose to, then asking for help is a gift that then allows others to contribute.

5. Gratitude celebration
Being thankful, appreciative and celebrating kindness is a gift to the giver and the receiver. You could be grateful for your health, family, job, friends, teachers, parents, siblings, music, passion, art, food, creativity, community, sleep, memories, home, sunrise, sunset or wisdom. Get the picture? Create and celebrate your own grateful list.

Celebrat*ion* Summary

- Take time to notice random acts of kindness.
- Be grateful to those who contribute to your life.
- Celebrate the people who bring joy and love to your life.
- Celebrate your life lessons, the good and the not so good. Both are your teachers.
- Celebrate the gift of today.

5 thoughtful ways to use your master-mind

8. Cognit*ion*

Quotation
Chance favours the prepared mind. – Louis Pasteur

Notation
Exercise your brain like you exercise your body. Mental, social, emotional, spiritual and physical health combine to make a well you. Remember, health is your wealth. To enhance cognition, and your ability to use your mind, find a field that interests you and challenges you. This helps to build on existing knowledge and acquire new knowledge and understanding.

The function of the brain is highly complex, as are the differing findings of what is best to 'train the brain.' If the workings of the human brain interest you, research this further. What could you choose to do to train this significant organ? What about a game, a puzzle, a crossword, a new language, hobby or dance?

Thrive on Five

1. Learn a new language

Join a class or group or use an app which gives you the opportunity to set a time limit of learning each day. Learn for your own interest, an upcoming holiday, or for work opportunities.

2. Learn a musical instrument

Music like all activities, sports, hobbies and interests has its own language. Learning something new requires the use of neural pathways and the language of music also has a personal connection. Children and adults alike can learn an instrument. If you could choose any instrument to learn, what would it be and why?

3. Non-dominant activity

Choose an activity you usually do with your dominant hand or foot and use your non-dominant hand or foot. Kick. Write. Draw. Eat. Initially it will feel unusual and you may find it difficult. This is because you are retraining the brain. Repeat this activity for a day, week or a month. Observe the changes.

4. Exercise

Exercise is important for overall wellbeing and benefits the body and mind. Regular exercise may help control hormone levels, reduce inflammation and stress, improve memory and thinking, and sleep patterns. Seek medical advice before starting any strenuous exercise. Exercise of the body and mind are beneficial at all ages and stages of development. Digital devices and apps can assist to monitor your progress. Be in motion.

5. Dance. Dance. Dance.

Dr Chris van Tulleken and Angela Rippon shared ageing studies in a BBC Documentary 2017, on *How to stay young, in body and mind*. The program shared the benefits of dancing to enhance not only physical wellbeing, but that remembering the dance routine assists brain function, and participation enhances social connections. You can dance alone, or socially with a partner or group. Perhaps join a class, a dance troupe, or just listen to the music of ABBA and be your own *Dancing Queen*, or King!

Cognit*ion* Summary

- Exercise your mind and body.
- Health is your wealth.
- Learn something new.
- Challenge yourself.
- What makes you a well-being?

5 views on treasure or trash

9. Collect*ion*

Quotation
To be human is to have a collection of memories that tells you who you are and how you got there. – Rosecrans Baldwin

Notation
Collections of physical things may have emotional attachments; therefore, collections are precious not only for any financial worth, but for the sentimental memories to a moment, a person, place and space in time. Like any collection, it is valuable to the owner, and to anyone else who for emotional, historical or valuable reasons, finds it interesting.

Thrive on Five

1. Interest or hobby collection

Have you or do you collect something for interest or as a hobby? Do you share your collection with others? Where do you keep your collection? Could you allow others to see it and perhaps raise money for a cause? Could you donate an object to a museum for others to visit the exhibit? Could you donate a piece to a charity for an auction to raise funds for an organisation close to your heart? Do you want to start a collection of something? Research any ideas you have. You may be surprised.

2. Donation collection

Could you volunteer your time or raise funds, or help a group, organisation, charity or a collective that assists others in need? Declutter and cleanse and you may find a collection of unused items that someone else may benefit from. Reduce. Reuse. Recycle.

3. Physical or digital collections

Visit museums, libraries and exhibitions near where you live or whilst on a holiday. You will be amazed at the collections that are available for public display. Ask a relative or friend do they know of an upcoming exhibition? Try something different, go to an event that perhaps you would not usually attend.

4. Create an exhibit

Are you an artist, photographer, sculptor, author, or collector of anything you think others may be interested to observe? Have you thought of exhibiting your work or collection at a café, restaurant, shop, public space or website? Could you earn an income from this? Could you give presentations about your collection to historical societies, museums, art galleries, organisations or interested groups? Could you write a book or an e-book about your collection or memories? Be imaginative.

5. Release and let go

Letting go of the emotional attachment to a collection may need to occur prior to the physical clearing. If you have ever wanted to release a collection of something, you will realise that knowing and then doing are two different processes. Realising is a start. Action achieves the results. Be kind to yourself. Ask for assistance. A valuable resource book pertaining to clutter clearing is: *Let it Go. Downsizing your Way to a Richer, Happier Life* by Peter Walsh.

Collect*ion* Summary

- Collect your thoughts before you speak or act in haste.
- Collections have attachments both positive and negative.
- Could you exhibit your collection?
- Could you share your collection, interest, hobby or talents?
- Childhood is a forever reference point, though it may be long past, it is not long forgotten.

5 ways to share your true essence

10. Communication

Quotation
Love is the only force capable of transforming an enemy into a friend. – Martin Luther King Jr

Notation
Communication conveys a message or information via words, pictures and actions. It is language and body language. It is sending and receiving a message and a way to connect. How often have you said something, and it landed the wrong way? Has your communication offended, not said enough, said too much, upset someone, been a joke at an inappropriate time, used the wrong words, inferred a different meaning to what was said, or body language did not match your words? Have you used words that did not match the dialogue in your head, or generally miscommunicated by your communication? You, me, everyone, has had one or more of these incidences occur.

Thrive on Five

1. Be mindful and heart full

Being mindful and heart full in your communication allows you to be clear, to say what there is to say, share clear boundaries for what you accept or do not accept, and it allows for the conveyance of a message or meaning. Be mindful of two way sharing. Communication has many forms. Words are what separate man from animal, either by spoken, written, digital or other mediums. Words are in different languages and symbols. Communication of love is the acceptance of yourself as you are and others how they are. Choose communication that unites, not divides and separates.

2. Attentive listening

Not new. But true. Humans have two ears for a reason and the art of listening is a skill never to be underestimated. By attentively listening to what the other person is sharing or asking, you can then respond appropriately. Respond to their need or request. Tune in and listen to your own inner voice. Tune into others and listen to what they are trying to share or teach. Listening is one powerful tool for lifetime learning.

3. Be confident

Speaking confidently in front of an audience ranks amongst the highest of fears. Being confident, being clear and being captivating are communication skills that assist with personal relationships and professional presentations. Being confident in you, and empathy for yourself and others, are keys to effective communication. Empowering yourself helps you to empower others and be of service, so that you can be a leader of your own life, and a leader in the world. Listen and learn from the advice from others but listen to your own guidance too.

4. Be empathic
Understanding or choosing to be compassionate of another's feelings is a prized skill and a generous gift. Being sensitive and being aware of another can provide care and comfort. Everyone is entitled to their opinion and you do not have to like it, but that is their opinion. Choosing when to say something, when to help or when to walk away is a skill. Some people like to engage in a battle of words and converse even when they know their point of view is incorrect, or do not believe in it. Be more compassionate to yourself and show genuine empathy to another. Communication is learning about what you can change and can't change and knowing the difference.

5. Be respectful
Be respectful of yourself and others. Be kind in the words you think, use and feel. Be kind in your actions. Thoughts, words and actions are all forms of communication to yourself and to others. Even when you think you are not communicating, you are. Try not to react to a situation. Breathe in love and act. Act in self-respect. Act in respect for others. Mother Teresa said, 'It's not how much we give, but how much love we put into the giving.'

Communication Summary
- Be respectful of yourself and others.
- Be kind to yourself and others.
- Be responsible for your thoughts, words and actions.

- Be proud of who you are.
- Be a leader in your life.

5 thoughtful ways to nourish your soul

11. Compan*ion*

Quotation
Valued companionships begin with a personal commitment to be an exemplary companion. – Joseph B Wirthlin

Notation
You are your lifetime companion. Have the best relationship with yourself by loving and accepting yourself for who you are, right now in the present moment.

Thrive on Five

1. Time as a companion

Your time is with many companions along life's journey. Make your time make a difference. Where could you offer your time and companionship, be it to a parent, friend, sibling, partner, relative, colleague, a child, an elderly citizen, an association, an animal, a hobby, interest, cause and of course for yourself? How could you take better care of yourself or someone you love?

2. Thoughts of companion

Your thoughts accompany you all the time. The type and kind of thoughts influence your words and actions. Be a friend to your thoughts not a stranger. Be a champion of kindness not darkness. Be an associate to your thoughts not an opponent. Be respectful of yourself. Saint Augustine said, 'Patience is the companion of wisdom.'

3. Children appreciate time

In my education and teaching experience, I observed children love to be with adults and appreciate the gift of time. To play is not just for children. Feel and observe the joy and laughter when adults allow their inner child to play and have fun. Where could you bring more play, joy and fun to your life or the life of a child? Kick autumn leaves. Jump in puddles. Roll down a hill. Laugh out loud. Children will remember the time you spend with them as the most precious gift.

4. Companion animals

Many different types of animals share lives with humans as companion or assistance animals. Having a pet is an enormous responsibility and commitment. Responsible ownership may include identification, registration and veterinary requirements and care. Regulations vary within states and countries. Assistance animals differ from pets and perform a specific service. They perform tasks and can help someone with an illness, disability or job. Could you or someone you know, benefit from a service pet or from being a responsible pet owner? Could you donate money or volunteer time to a companion animal organisation, to assist others in need?

5. Companion for the elderly

Growing older is inevitable. In this transient world, not everyone has family close by, is able to care for themselves, has physical mobility, or access to transport. Is there someone in your family, neighbourhood or community that would benefit from your gift of time, companionship, listening ear, or assistance? Simple things mean a lot. You could mow the lawn, take them shopping, cook a meal or share a conversation. How could you be of service?

Compan*ion* Summary

- You are your life companion. Be kind in your thoughts, words and actions.
- A child is within. Remember to play, laugh and be joyous.
- Be kind to all people of all generations.
- How could you help a companion/assistance animal organisation?
- As time goes by, let time be your friend.

5 nurturing viewpoints of self and others

12. Compass*ion*

Quotation
If you want others to be happy, practice compassion. If you want to be happy, practice compassion. – Dalai Lama

Notation
As the Dalai Lama points out, at the heart of compassion is compassion of your own heart. Demonstrate kindness, caring and a willingness to help others. Everyone is dealing with something or a misfortune and Maya Angelou sums this up, 'My mission in life is not merely to survive, but to thrive; and to do so with some passion, some compassion, some humour, and some style.'

Thrive on Five

1. Self-compassion
Be kind to yourself. At any moment in time things happen that can make you reflect on life. The loss of a loved one, a job, a dream, a pet, or anything you are dealing with, needs to be grieved. Loss is grief, it opens things that were closed, or it closes things that were open. Whatever it is and however it affects you is different from someone else. Be compassionate and stop judging yourself. Seek out any assistance you may need. Be kind to yourself. Give yourself time to be there for yourself and allow whatever is surfacing to be healed. Healing requires you to nurture your body, mind, heart and soul, and take time for you.

2. Compassion for others. Be kind to others.
We all deal with things differently. Expecting others to deal with something as you would, imposes your opinions and judgements and at a time of crisis this may not be helpful. Wanting to solve a hurt is a natural human reaction, to take the pain away, to share the burden or the load. Often a listening ear, without the offer of problem solving and without judgement, are gifts of energy and time that are priceless. Being kind, truly is a gift to you and to the person receiving this gift.

3. Loss of a pet
To some, a pet is like family. Be considerate of yourself or people who have pet babies. These connections are an energy relationship with another living creature. Take time to deal with the grief and loss. Be kind.

4. Loss of a dream

Many people's dreams are unfulfilled for whatever reason and some people's dream may never be realised. This may cause grief at the loss. For some dreams, no matter what someone says, the loss can never ever be replaced, or the dream fulfilled. Time, reframing and reflection can help healing. Learning to be present and grateful for everything in your life, each moment and each day, is the gift of being present. Your life is a precious gift and is about coming from heart and filling your heart with that which makes it sing. What is that for you?

5. Ask for help

Have compassion for yourself. Put your hand up and share when circumstances are not okay for you. When you need assistance, support, a helping hand, a change or have a request, ask. People you love, live or work with can help when you share what you are able to and unable to do. Asking allows others to contribute to your life.

Compass*ion* Summary

- At the heart of compassion is the compassion of your heart.
- Be compassionate and kind to yourself.
- Be compassionate towards others. We all have lessons to learn.
- Live your life and create your dreams and goals.
- Asking for help is a strength not a weakness, and it allows others to contribute as you would for them.

5 ways to express success and happiness

13. Congratulation

Quotation
May today's success be the beginning of tomorrow's achievements. Congratulations. – Author Unknown

Notation
Do you remember the last time you had a special occasion, giving good wishes and compliments to someone, or receiving them from family, friends, colleagues or peers? Do you remember the joy of celebrating that good fortune, success, efforts and discoveries? Do you celebrate success, or do you just move onto something else? Life offers many opportunities to be congratulated and offer congratulations. In those moments, pause and reflect on the time and effort spent on a cause, project, skill, or acquisition of knowledge. Pause to learn, to teach, to understand, to be present to the magnificence that you are, and that of those around you. Congratulate yourself or someone else, on the small steps to mastery, as well as the mastering of the concept or completion of the task or project.

Thrive on Five

1. Acknowledge someone

Express your congratulations and share your joy and happiness for someone's achievement in their personal life, or the contribution to your life or the lives of others. Observe where and how people not only believe and achieve, but have a remarkable way of enhancing others' lives, and making the world a more joyous place. Who could you acknowledge, recommend, congratulate or even nominate for an award? Notice and appreciate the small acts of kindness around you all the time. Be grateful and thankful for these acts.

2. Self-congratulations

Do you need a little self-congratulation? Have you ever started a new venture or project and it was difficult, but you persevered with positivity and completed it? Often deeds and actions you do and give may seemingly go unnoticed, but the true essence of giving is without expectation. Congratulate yourself for all the little things that contribute to the big things. You deserve happiness, health and success. Remember things come back to you in many ways and perhaps not from the person you give to.

3. Congratulations celebration

Who could you organise a celebration for? Who deserves to be recognised? Gather together in known anticipation or in surprise, and honour someone for their contribution to your life, the lives of others, or for their achievement. Public acknowledgement allows for others to contribute and then share the impact of someone else's success and achievement. There are a lot of generous, compassionate, helpful, unassuming, kind souls who donate time and energy without expectation of anything. A grateful and heartfelt thank you is deserved. Make a diary of birthdays and anniversaries for family and friends and celebrate your loved ones.

4. Congratulations on the journey
There is no destination, just the journey. Lao Tzu said, 'A journey of a thousand miles begins with a single step.' Encourage and acknowledge yourself and others along the way, be constructive and give praise where necessary. Congratulate yourself for each part of the journey. Start. Take one step at a time, just start, and as this unknown author wrote, 'Turn your life into cans and your dreams into plans.'

5. Creative Congratulations
There are many reasons for congratulations and many ways to express it. To make it specific, relevant and personal, you could use a different language, an inspiring quote, create a poem or song. Send a text, email, card or call. Be creative and surprise someone deserving your congratulations.

Congratulat*ion* Summary
- Acknowledge and celebrate your achievements.
- Celebrate the success and happiness of loved ones.
- Who could you organise a celebration for?
- Celebrating allows you to bring together in one place those you love.
- Celebrate the steps to achievement as well as the achievement itself.

5 relationship views of self, others and the universe

14. Connect*ion*

Quotation
Connection to self, to others, to nature and to the universe is the relationship of interconnection. – Raelene Dal Santo

Notation
Who and what are you connected to? Connection is a reminder that when you feel a disconnect to someone or something then it is a reminder to go within, to ground yourself physically and spiritually. Connect to yourself and be present to perhaps what the disconnect is. Forgiveness is always the key. Forgive yourself and forgive others. It is a freeing gift that you not only deserve but need. Be guided by this Louise Hay affirmation, 'I love and approve of myself.' Repeat it to yourself hundreds of times a day. Being present to what is in your life is grounding, connecting you to the abundance that is already present. Reunite yourself with you.

Thrive on Five

1. The '*ion*' word with a difference

Of all the *'ion'* words used in this book, this one encompasses them all. It is the one word that may make the biggest difference to yourself and the lives of those you love. Connectedness to yourself and to one another not only physically but psychologically, are the love threads that unite the world. Connection occurs on many levels. These being personal, local and global. When we connect with ourselves and others, it allows for the betterment of all. It allows you to feel a sense of belonging. It allows you to see and feel the interrelatedness of humanity. By connecting and collaborating, there is a victory on many levels for an individual, for an organisation and for communities. What is today's connection for you?

2. Family connect

Is there a member of your family for whatever reason, you do not associate with? Is there someone in your family that could benefit from an olive branch, helping to rebuild the family tree. Could you be that person who forgives and extends the branch to build or rebuild connections? Forgiveness is a gift to the giver as well as the receiver.

3. Volunteer to bring near

Is there a community organisation or group that would benefit from your time and energy to help others? If you are unable to make a daily, weekly or monthly commitment, is there a seasonal event or festive celebration where you could give your time? Read papers, magazines, search online or ask local organisations for avenues where you could assist.

4. Connect to self

Is there a yoga, Tai Chi, Qi Gong or meditation class you could try? These types of physical pursuits allow for breath work and help to create a peaceful, calm and meditative state that allows connection to self and to the universe. This connection allows you to go within and to be an observer of self.

5. Like attracts like

Is there a pursuit that you are passionate about? If you research, you will discover that others somewhere in the world are passionate about it too. Connecting with people of a similar ilk allows for: social connectedness, learning and teaching, the spark of an idea, and problem solving. It may give you the opportunity to participate in an event to move towards your goal or create newness in your chosen passion. What have you always wanted to try or be? Seek it. Be it. Do it.

Connect*ion* Summary

- Being grateful reminds you of connectedness.
- Connectedness is the love thread that unites the world. (I love this.)
- Do you know anyone who may need an olive branch?
- How can you offer your time and energy to a volunteer organisation?
- Like attracts like. Find your tribe and vibe.

5 observances of human connectedness

15. Consump*tion*

Quotation
Infinite growth of material consumption in a finite world is an impossibility.
– E F Schumacher

Notation
Consumption depends on the product and the availability, access and cost of that product to the consumer. Consumption of products is not the sole type, it could be of information, energisation or communication. Everyone is a consumer. A consumer of something you need for basic survival, or as a want.

Thrive on Five

1. Global consumption of resources

Is what the consumer is told, fed or shown, cause for inclusion or exclusion. Like everything in life, perception is key and yours and someone else's may be similar or no correlation between. Humans are continually creating new products, creating industry and markets, for both needs and wants. Mindful production and mindful consumption may be keys to minimisation of wasted or finite resources. How can you monitor your use of resources so there is sustainability?

2. Food consumption as energy

Humans attain chemical energy from food, and food sustains metabolism. What foods are you consuming as a source of fuel for your body, mind and soul? Daily life and seasons give you choices and the type of food to eat. This is determined by financial, physically accessible, and personal preferences. Are you aware of the nutritional value of the foods you consume for optimal health? Does the food you eat give your body energy and allow you to attain and maintain good health? What is one food changing habit you could add or delete for your body, mind and soul? Learn how to interpret food labels and note the hidden ingredients in some food preparations.

3. Information: factual, fake or fantasy

The consumption of information has many forms in the digital era. Social media generates news that trends on a range of issues. Individuals can influence a populous as well as corporations, on a national and international stage. This is the creation and consumption of national and global cultures. With the ever-accessible world, is satisfaction via consumption increasing for humans? Is consumption affecting happiness and living a life you love with purpose and passion increasing? Is life a joy? Questions to muse and ponder on how digital information affects consumption and emotions, both positive and negative.

4. Energy as power consumption

Energy and its forms are many as discussed in Energisation. Access to energy means opportunities for nations and individuals. In your household, there are always ways you can reduce the energy used. Examples could include: minimise possessions, use the sun and wind to dry clothes, plant a tree, compost, garden, turning off appliances when not in use, reduce the number of consumer products, recycle products into something else and reusing where possible. National and global campaigns champion individuals and organisations to reduce the consumption of energy. How could you play your part?

5. Global access and business

Niche businesses have global audiences. Do you have an idea, product or service that could be focused and harnessed to reach millions? Once upon a time, only corporations had the resources to access large populations; individuals now have access to the resources to access global populations. Do you have an idea, a passion, a cause or a purpose that awaits a global audience? What solution to a problem do you have to share with the world?

Consump*tion* Summary

- Consumption on many levels, is within and around you all the time.

- Food consumption sustains metabolism.
- Be mindful and heart full of the information you consume and share.
- How could you conserve energy consumption in your environments?
- How could you utilise the digital revolution to enhance your lifestyle, cause or business?

5 unifying reminders of human difference yet sameness

16. Cooperat*ion*

Quotation
In union, there is strength. – Aesop

Notation
Working together for a common goal or reason is the act of cooperation. Being cooperative is the support, contribution or helpfulness that makes relationships work. It does not mean giving in, rather being supportive and assisting with requests where and how you can. Working collaboratively and co-operatively allows for teamwork and mutual associations. This may not be easy but a way to collaboration and a win/win negotiation.

Thrive on Five

1. Six degrees, or is it?

All humans are here on Earth for a reason. Some may feel they know or realise their purpose, and others are on the journey of discovery. With free will, sometimes even when you feel you know, you may then choose to change. Whatever the circumstances, our daily lives are interconnected with other humans for our wellbeing, whether they are known to you or not.

2. Interdependence

Food supply, transport, sanitation, health, education, business and industry are but a few of the areas humans are interdependent. The more you connect with this link to another, the more you realise cooperation is inextricably essential for both receiving and giving. With understanding and compassion, in what conversations and situations could you demonstrate cooperation?

3. Firewood and Fires

Not everyone has the viewpoint of cooperation. Some have the expectations of subordination. Empathy levels vary. Your expectation of others, or someone co-operating, may not happen. You choose what works for you and only you will know when it is time to stay, or time to give your energy to another situation, relationship, cause or project. Although you may not light a fire for warmth or power in this age of technology, this Chinese proverb summaries unity, 'Only when all contribute their firewood can they build up a strong fire.' What or who in your life ignites joy? What or who makes you feel stagnant and needs releasing? How will cooperation benefit your needs or wants?

4. Human commonality
Whoever you Are, by Mem Fox is one of my favourite children's books. Its message is to teach and learn, that no matter what physical and cultural differences appear on the exterior of a person, the interior part of humans is the same. With empathy and compassion, you learn that connectedness and interconnectedness unite. Bill Clinton said, 'We all do better when we work together. Our differences do matter, but our common humanity matters more.' Remember all humanity is linked and interdependent. Cooperation enhances our participation in life.

5. Progress and Success
All humans are on a life journey. Some love their path, some take it as it comes, some love direction, some stay on path when it no longer serves. Wherever you are at, remember it is a moment in time, and this moment does not define the next moment, nor your tomorrow. You are bigger than whatever you perceive as an error. Making anew, requires honesty, strength, courage and integrity. Words perhaps, but their display in action, like the smallest act of kindness are welcomed, noticed and appreciated. Henry Ford, sums this up, 'Coming together is a beginning, staying together is progress, and working together is success.'

Cooperation Summary
- Teamwork and mutual respect are well respected.
- Humans daily lives are interconnected.

- What enhances cooperation in your life?
- Cooperation is the thread that unites individuals.
- Relationships need cooperation.

5 ways to discover creativity within and around you

17. Creat*ion*

Quotation
If you think you can do a thing or think you can't do a thing, you're right.
– Henry Ford

Notation
In this sense, I am referring to the creation that you are and the creativity inside of you and from you. These include: the inception of an idea, the formation of something in the physical world, your imagination, and the foundation or the production of something.

I grew up on farms, and nature has a way of teaching and reminding you of the creation and the cycle of life. Some surprisingly beautiful, some harsh and sad. Life on the land was a positive learning experience full of loving memories. The farm taught me the fragility of life, the preciousness of food and water, and teamwork needed in life.

Thrive on Five

1. Your creativity
The universe is full of inventions, concoctions, handiwork, performances, items and ideas. What is it that you enjoy for your creativity to exist and bloom? Do you allow yourself the time to birth ideas and products, be creative, play, innovate, imagine, and be calm and centred? What is your creative outlet?

2. Try something different
People naturally gravitate to what best suits them. Your lifestyle and how you choose to live is your preference. Perhaps to spark creativity, try something different. Drive a different way to work. Read a different genre that you would not usually read. Bake a different recipe from familiar foods. Listen to music of your childhood. Just try unfamiliar instead of familiar. Be surprised by your insights. Try something new.

3. Inside or Outside activities
If you like to be outside, try being inside, and vice versa. Learn something new. Being engaged in an activity you love and are passionate about, brings joy and may spark new creative directions. Write down any activity you love to do or would like to do. Write all the things you know or would like to know about that activity. How could you access this information? Who could or would you like to speak with regarding this activity? What other industries or services are associated with this activity? Be surprised at the insights and creativity this activity may spark.

4. Imagination
In times of silence or activity, listening or speaking, learning or

teaching, an idea may arise. A thought, image, or word may spark your imagination, trigger intention, then action. When people choose to change their life, or create something, I like to ask these questions: What or who is your inspiration? What was the spark that ignited the passion? What did you learn? Listen to your inner voice that always guides you. Write down your thoughts or answers and upon reflection, you may gain more insights.

5. Nature
Nature has a great way of grounding, nurturing, inspiring and reminding you of daily life. It teaches you. It nurtures you. Nature creates the ebbs and flows in the rivers and oceans, the sunrise and sunset of the day and night, the waxing and waning of the moon, the changing of the seasons in the world and in your world. Spend time in nature. Notice Mother nature's lessons.

Creat*ion* Summary

- Share your 'younique' talents with the world.
- Tick the bucket list and try something that you have always wanted to.
- Newness allows creativity to shine.
- Create time to create newness.
- Nature grounds you and reminds of the fragility and beauty of life.

5 nurturing ways to release what no longer serves you

18. Detoxification

Quotation

If you don't take care of this the most magnificent machine that you will ever be given…where are you going to live? – Karyn Calabrese

Notation

Detoxification refers to the process of removing toxicity from something. Be it substances, thoughts, people or things. It is making it less harmful to you, someone else or something. What or who do you need to detox from? Could you eliminate any of the following that do not serve your health, healing or wellbeing: stimulants, drugs, alcohol, refined sugars, saturated fats, use of cleaning chemicals, chemicals within food or products you consume, or stress. Ralph Waldo Emerson's quote is apt, 'The first wealth is health.'

Thrive on Five

1. Detoxify your body
Is there a substance that is toxic for you? A medical or health care provider may suggest you detoxify your body from a substance. Tune into your own inner wisdom to guide you. This process of elimination of toxins from the body will vary for everyone. Who or what could you turn to for assistance?

2. Foods that detox your body
Socrates said, 'Let food be thy medicine and medicine be thy food.' The body eliminates toxins through the kidneys, intestines, skin, lymphatic system and the lungs. Detoxification or cleansing of the blood is done by the liver. Nutrition is one way that assists the body to nourish, renew and cleanse. It assists to gain and maintain optimum health. Individual medical or health care needs vary. Tune into your inner wisdom. Consult with a medical or health provider if required.

3. Detox your thoughts
Louise Hay dedicated her life to teaching the power of positive affirmations and how the point of your power is always in the present moment. My favourite book by her is, *The Power is Within You*. I read this as a young adult, and am forever reminded of the power of words, whether spoken, written, or as thoughts. Words are powerful tools that can unite or divide. How do you use your words, to yourself or to others? Are they disempowering or empowering?

4. What is your detox style
What do you need to detox? Do you need a food detox, a person detox, thoughts detox, stress detox, digital detox or

clutter detox? How could you reduce stress? What is one thing that you could do today that would make a difference to your life? What activities could you choose to enhance your wellbeing? Remember, one day at a time, as life occurs, one day at a time. Who or what brings joy to your life? Breathe and breathe. Allow oxygen to circulate through your body. What is one positive thing you could do for yourself today? Ask for help where you need it and allow others to contribute to your life. Allow yourself to receive the gifts that others offer to your life.

5. Mind/Body connection
Healing your body from the inside out is the aim of detoxification. Cleansing and nourishing the body can help you attain and maintain optimal health. You will discover your preferred way to help your body achieve this aim. The impact of stress can never be underestimated. Find ways to relax and reset mental thoughts and reactions to balance wellbeing of mind and body.

Detoxification Summary

- Your health is your most valuable asset.
- What or who do you need to detox?
- Seek medical or health care assistance if required.
- Nurture your body with nutritional food and your mind with kind thoughts.
- What is one lifestyle changing choice you could make today?

LIVE WITH LOVE

5 thoughts on choosing what matters to you

19. Direct*ion*

Quotation
There is no greater agony than bearing an untold story inside of you. – Maya Angelou

Notation
Everyone needs help with direction at some stage of life. The orange light may seem to continually flash, and you become uncertain of what to do, have or be. You feel stuck, with no motion and no direction. The internal GPS (Geographical Positioning System) is not calibrating and the universe seemingly not aligning either. Tune into your inner guidance for direction.

Thrive on Five

1. Patience

You will find direction, you will find your purpose, you will find your passion, you will get the opportunity and the right people at the right time will be in your life. It may be negative or positive. Take the lesson. Take the opportunity. Be courageous and tell your story to yourself and share it with the world. Everyone is on their own journey and has stories affecting their life. Be patient with yourself and being a patient listener, you may also help someone else find their direction. Dream and act. Create and live the life you love.

2. You are not lost

If you feel lost, are dealing with grief, loss or trauma, Helen Keller reminds us, 'What we have once enjoyed we can never lose. All that we love deeply becomes a part of us.' You are not lost, but it can feel that way. To change direction or try out a new path, you may need support and guidance. Someone will be there to support you, to help you. The universe will provide. Reaching out and asking for help is not a weakness, it is kindness to yourself and it allows others to contribute to your life, as you would for them. Ask. Someone will be there to give direction, then allow yourself to receive. Kindness is a gift. Enjoy its presence.

3. What really counts?

Here are some words of wisdom form Albert Einstein, 'Not everything that can be counted counts, and not everything that counts can be counted.' Have you ever stopped and thought about what really matters to you? Really, really? What are your values? Have your values shifted? Are you living a life that you love or just following a direction you thought you 'should'? Is something, someone, or you, holding 'younique' you back from achieving your goals and dreams. *Live with Love* and joy.

4. Be prepared and progress
The purpose of writing this book is to help 'younique' you, the reader, live your dreams. My hope is that the life you want to live inside you is fulfilled and that you find a way to allow that inner you to shine in your world, and the world. You will have fears. You will need to be resilient. You may need to shift focus or reframe thoughts and attitudes to follow your dream. Sometimes it may feel people may not understand or like your choices, but they love you for who you are and who you will become. It is best to live life with fear, then to be fearful of never living your life. Love will always, always, be stronger than fear. Love yourself.

5. Proceed with kindness
Mark Twain, shared these words, 'Kindness is the language which the deaf can hear and the blind can see.' Kindness is the best place to come from, but sometimes a difficult road to travel. With any relationship, only you will know what direction to go; when it is best to stop going down a road, to proceed with caution, or to keep going. Ask for personal or professional help if needed. Despite what the road is like, it is best to proceed with kind words and kind deeds. The universe has a way of taking care of you, and even though kindness may not always be visible or tangible, it really is both. Notice kindness. Be kindness.

Direct*ion* Summary

- Live the life that yearns to be lived.
- People, circumstances and opportunities to assist you realise your dream are always around you.
- Observe kindness.
- Who or what really matters in your life?
- Be kindness.

5 benefits of teaching and learning

20. Education

Quotation

Education is the most powerful weapon which you can use to change the world. – Nelson Mandela

Notation

'Sometimes in life we do not only need a transformation we need a revolution,' is a quote by an unknown author. Choose to enhance your qualifications in a current occupation, career or job. Or, you may as the quote suggests, choose to revolutionise your life and retrain in an industry, profession or interest, that is totally different from what you currently know. Education provides instruction and facilitation to enlighten lifelong learning opportunities.

Thrive on Five

1. Believe in yourself

Stop limiting yourself and remember the saying, 'Where there is a will there is a way.' You will find the strength, courage and resources both physical and financial, to enable you to choose a change. What have you always wanted to learn, study or be? Be it. As George Michaels's eighties T-shirt shouted, 'Choose Life!' Choose what you want and find a way. Search, inquire and ask for guidance. Listen to your own wisdom and learn from the wisdom of others. Plan. Create. Enjoy.

2. Learn something new

Learn something new, such as a language, craft, sport, instrument or dance. A new activity may use different words, symbols or materials, giving you and your mind access to newness, and therefore extend learning.

3. Volunteer

Volunteer your time and energy to teach others something new or support them in a field where you get to use and share your skills, experiences, knowledge and talents. Someone will always need what you offer and share.

4. Social connectedness

Find a course or activity that interests you. This could be a community course, learning a skill from a loved one, or asking for guidance from someone you respect. Not only do you learn, gain new skills and knowledge, you also create personal or professional networks. Human interconnectedness is vital for wellbeing.

5. Learn and work online

The digital world offers opportunities to learn, teach and connect. Many organisations realise this and create situations so that people can virtually attend, participate and contribute, without being physically present. This provides immediate access regardless of distance. It reduces costs and allows for other life commitments. Do you want to be your own boss? What business could you create?

Education Summary

- Connect with like-minded people.
- Offer your time, energy, knowledge or skills to a volunteer organisation.
- Be open to learning. Be open to teaching and sharing knowledge and skills.
- Education develops potential.
- Learning is a lifelong skill.

5 recharging ways to energise your life

21. Energisation

Quotation
We are all connected; To each other, biologically. To the earth, chemically. To the rest of the universe atomically. – Neil de Grasse Tyson

Notation
Albert Einstein said, 'Everything in life is vibration.' The ebb and flow of energy between people, around people, around the universe, is immeasurable and omnipresent. Many people are sensitive to others energy and the energy around them. It can be overwhelming at times, but it also highlights their ability to show empathy towards others and be helpful in their re-energisation.

Thrive on Five

1. Types of energy

There is much research about energy in relationships and types of energy. These types include: chemical, biological, anatomical, magnetic, light, gravitational, electrical, sound, nuclear, kinetic and heat. What are your energy observations and experiences in your relationships with people and the environment?

2. Energy within

Energy can fluctuate daily. If you keep a diary for a month noticing how you feel each day, even at different times of one day, you would notice that you use a variety of words perhaps from powered to drained. Energy is something we feel, and you do not need scientific devices to describe how you feel. Many philosophies around the world describe the energy fields within and around us. These include but are not exclusive to: Ruwach or Chay (Hebrew), Chi or Qi (Taoism), Spiritus (Latin), Pneuma and Psyche (Greek), Shakti and Kundalini (Hindu), Prana (Sanskrit). These fields of energy descriptions may provide you interesting reading.

Food is a source of energy for the body and the types you consume can affect you. Monitor your energy levels. Notice how it affects you and those around you. Protect your energy by reviewing your communication and connection.

3. Energy between people

The flow of energy we feel within, can also be felt between people. Although you may not understand it, you can be affected by it. Generally, it is a vibrating energy feeling, described with positive or negative words. Positivity vibrates and emanates from some people. Some people give you energy. You will know this instantly. You will be energised and enthused by it. On the other hand, some feel like they drain it. A bit like emotional vampires. These people may put you a little off centre and other people really shake your energy around, and you could feel unsettled. Sometimes you can see it or hear it, in verbal and nonverbal communication. Energy can either attract or it can repel. Some people can feel this energy either in someone's company or from a distance, whilst others may not feel this interpersonal energy. Can you feel this energy between people?

4. Sustainable energy

Types of energy used in the world to generate power vary, depending on geographical location, government regulations and personal access and preference. These energy types include: solar, wave, nuclear, wind, hydroelectric, biomass, geothermal, hydrogen, tidal, and fossil fuels (oil, natural gas and coal). There are arguments, discussions and legislations advocating the best power type, energy consumption and energy renewal. Energy provides power both in the physical and financial sense. It is of personal, national and global interest. How do you use power? Are you aware of what and how you consume energy? How could you conserve energy use? What energy issues concern you?

5. Universal energy

Energy affects our daily lives, from the energy within and from the environments in which you live. Nikola Tesla said, 'If you want to find the secrets of the universe, think in terms of energy, frequency and vibration.' Energy may not be visible, but its effects are. What gives you energy? How do you share your energy with the universe? I am referring to your 'younique' gifts and latent potential awaiting to shine. Let your energy shine.

Energisat*ion* Summary

- Humanity is interconnected.
- Energy may not be visible but its effects will be.
- Your energy changes daily.
- Energy influences your life.
- Energy is essential to life.

5 ways to discover your 'love made visible' to the world

22. Express*ion*

Quotation
It is the supreme art of the teacher to awaken joy in creative expression and knowledge. – Albert Einstein

Notation
There are many forms of expression, of knowledge and of love. To awaken that which is yearning, and to then practice it, can be desire fulfilled. A sense of contentment. The process of learning, creating and then sharing, is an expression of who you are to yourself, to your world and to the world. This expression could be your voice, your craft, your talents, your skills, your knowledge, your generosity of spirit or your creativity. For political, cultural, civil, or personal reasons, this gift is not afforded to everyone, yet a gift that is inside everyone.

Thrive on Five

1. Food as an expression of love

For me, and perhaps for you, Maya Angelou's words are apt, 'I'm just someone who likes cooking and for whom sharing food is a form of expression.' To some, cooking and baking food, is 'love made visible.' What I love about food is that it unites and brings people together for conversation, celebration and at times commemoration. Eating unties humanity. The what, how, where, who, when and why may differ but the eating unites. What new or traditional food could you cook or bake? Who could you invite to share or prepare a meal and connect with conversation and joy?

2. Your voice

Your ability to say what there is to say for you and your life, is the biggest gift you can give to yourself. To speak up, to stand up, to stand out and stand proud is not easy and even overwhelming at times. When you are courageous and strong and speak your truth, you find even more courage and strength and support than you knew could exist. Like most things in life, taking one action towards your dream, goal or truth and then the next, despite the fear, you move closer and closer towards it. Remember the journey of life is a process, there is no product nor destination. Enjoy it. What is one action you could take today that would move you closer to your dreams or goals?

3. Allow your humanity to shine

Have you ever noticed that you are most happy, calm or at peace when you can express your creativity, sometimes as an escape, sometimes ever present? Allow your vision to be your expression. Let your radiance, beauty, grace, talents, calmness, kindness, gentleness, strength, courage, love, sensitivity, confidence, hope, dignity, generosity, integrity, humility, essence and even goofiness shine and shine brightly, as an expression of who you are, and who you know yourself to be. Shine like a lighthouse. Shine. Shine. Shine.

4. Express yourself

Express the essence of who you are. Find what gives you pleasure and is a creative expression of 'younique' you. Run, play, skip, hop, dance, draw, paint, write, garden, sing, create music, solve problems, be sensitive, construct, or whatever you choose to do and be. Find something that allows you to express your individuality. Allow it and you, to shine.

5. Expression in Communication

Freedom of expression is a basic human right but is not always afforded to everyone. The act of expressing your thoughts and feelings using verbal and nonverbal communication allows for sharing of emotions. This communication allows for and enhances the wellbeing of a human being. What is it you need or want to express in your communication?

Express*ion* Summary

- Express your creativity.
- What is your 'love made visible?'
- Allow your humanity to shine.
- Express your 'youniqueness.'
- Speak up. Stand up. Stand out.

5 ways to express your individuality

23. Fash*ion*

Quotation
Every day is a fashion show and the world is the runway. – Coco Chanel

Notation
'Fashion' in terms of style, behaviour or decoration is individual. To construct, design, build or create something is individual. Influences of culture, trends, availability of natural, physical and financial resources vary. Like art and beauty, fashion interpretation and appreciation is in the eyes of the beholder. Someone may like it, or not. That is okay. Each to their own.

Thrive on Five

1. Clothing fashion

Clothing is a covering. It can be a basic need to protect the body from the elements of nature, from danger, or to cover the body in a social context for personal, professional, religious, cultural or celebratory reasons. Do you have excess, unwanted or unused clothes that you could sell, donate to a charity or give to someone?

2. Individual fashion

The way you dress, decorate your home, or the behaviours you present, are all part of the individual 'fashion' that is 'younique' you. Preference of colours, textures, fabrics, materials, positioning, economics, nature, sustainability, places and people may influence your style. Research, read magazines, visit open homes and gardens to discover a style you like. Be be-you-ti-ful you.

3. Your creative fashion in the world

Do you like design? Do you like to create? Do you like to build? Careers in 'fashion' vary and could include the clothing, imaging and styling industry, architecture, photography, gardening, landscaping, arts, crafts, interior design, engineering, building, automotive, coding, music and theatre production. If you would like a change in career or just interested in learning what occupations use your 'younique' talents, a suggested read is, *What Colour is Your Parachute?* by Richard N Bolles. What activity could you do, to use design thinking, to create something aesthetic or functional?

4. Design fashion

If you think about it, thinking, thinking, you are designing in thoughts, words and actions all the time. Humans are devising and designing all the time: changing existing situations into preferred situations, designing processes to improve experiences, needs and services of individual and communities. Coco Chanel refers to the world as a fashion runway. What could you design to change your world, or the world of someone else?

5. Technology fashion

The skills, techniques, goods and services, and inventions created by technology influence lifestyle. Individuals and businesses use these tools to create and develop more products and services. The ever-accessible world allows for specific niche markets to be created and catered for. How do you utilise technology in your life?

Fash*ion* Summary

- Humans are continually designing, influencing and creating.
- Fashion, like any area of life, is individual.
- Individual fashion in any field of life allows for your 'youniqueness' to shine.
- Humans are in a constant design of thoughts, words and actions.
- Fashion is another word for trends, and this encompasses all aspects of lifestyle.

5 respectful ways of generational teaching and learning

24. Generat*ion*

Quotation
Each generation imagines itself to be more intelligent than the one that went before it, and wiser than the one that comes after it. – George Orwell

Notation
Sharing and learning is the essence of what forms generations. One is not better than before or after, but perception can be otherwise. Being kind and respectful of others, and of where you are at, would help the world be a better place and this is what each generation would like another to realise.

Thrive on Five

1. Positive generation

To make a positive difference in the world, to find solutions to problems instead of passing them on, is perhaps a responsible goal. You can only be responsible for you, and if everyone did this, then the world itself would be more positive for the next generation. What could you learn from or teach someone from another generation?

2. Peaceful generation

Peace occurs on many levels. It is within and the feeling from around in your immediate world, then nationally and globally. If peace is being tranquil within and free from conflict around, is your world, and the world peaceful? What is peace to you? How do you remain peaceful within, when all around you is not harmonious, even hostile? How could you create a peaceful solution in your relationships, organisations or community? A sense of calm is a true gift. How do you create peace within?

3. Sustainable generation

If sustaining something is maintaining it at a certain level, over time, what are you committed to upholding, defending or conserving? Over time periods things change, ideas change, weather changes, life changes and people change. Impacts on people and nature is a result of change and minimising destructive change on the environment, organisations and people, is an ideal of sustainability. What this is and how it is achieved, is of continual world-wide discussion of generations, of governments and its citizens. What could you reduce, reuse or recycle in your world? What causes are you passionate about sustaining and maintaining for yourself and others?

4. Caring generation

An attitude of caring for other human beings no matter their age or stage is a true gift to the receiver. As Dr David R Hamilton, author of *The Five Side Effects of Kindness*, shares in his words and writing: the practice of kindness for others, also benefits the giver. This practice of concern and generosity towards others does not go unnoticed by the universe. Sometimes, people are for whatever reason needing care, acts of compassion, grace and understanding. The gifts of time and love are priceless. Kindness begets kindness. Be kind to yourself and others.

5. Change generation

Do you like things to stay the same or do you like change? The world is ever changing, ever transient, and daily you are reminded of different things happening in the world. Things are altering and modifying and what was, seems either new and refreshing, or different and overwhelming. What is something you would like to stay the same and what is something you would like to be different? This is different for every individual and navigating change, is a daily practice. Change happens within and around you every moment. Be kind as you navigate change.

Generat*ion* Summary

- Sharing and learning is uniting.
- How do you create calm and peace within and around you?
- Acts of compassion, grace, understanding and kindness never go unnoticed by the universe.

LIVE WITH LOVE

- Kindness is love made visible.
- Navigating change is a daily practice.

5 thoughts why water is liquid gold

25. Hydrat*ion*

Quotation
Water is the most neglected nutrient in your diet, but one of the most vital.
– Julia Child

Notation
Water makes up a large percentage of the Earth's surface. Water also makes up a large percentage of the human body. It is essential to sustain life.

Thrive on Five

1. Hydration

When and how much water to drink is an individual choice. Besides being an essential requirement for overall health and wellbeing, water may help to boost energy, improve mood, enhance concentration and aid digestion. Is your body hydrated for optimum health?

2. Dehydration

Not having adequate water for optimum health is dehydration. This can result in lack of concentration, fatigue, headaches and severe medical conditions. Thirst can be a sign of dehydration as is the colour of your urine. Some foods and drinks are diuretics causing you to pass extra fluids. As with everything, everybody is different. Do you need reminders to drink water and hydrate?

3. Remind children to drink

The provision of, and access to clean drinking water can assist to regulate body temperature, calm, and improve body function. Children live mostly in the present and often need reminders to drink, to replenish from play, from both mental and physical activities. All humans need hydration and access to clean drinking water and sanitation. How could you conserve water in your environment?

4. Safe and unsafe drinking water

The issue of the access and provision of clean drinking water and sanitation is a worldwide health and societal issue of inequality. Many local, national and global organisations aim to address this issue for billions of people across the world. Is there an organisation you could support with time or finances that would enable this most precious resource, to be accessible to fellow human beings?

5. Protection of water sources
The protection of ground water is important to individuals and to nations. Protection from contamination is the aim, to provide access to fresh supplies. Collaboration by governments, scientists, farmers and consumers all united, is the key for the protection of safe drinking water, run off and sanitation. What could you do to ensure this is created or sustained on a local, national or global level? What skills or ideas do you have to contribute to water containment or conservation?

Hydrat*ion* Summary
- Water is essential for life.
- Water is health and wealth.
- Are you adequately hydrated for optimal health and wellbeing?
- Remind children to hydrate.
- Conserve water, a valuable life sustaining ingredient.

5 thoughtful ways of interacting

26. Impress*ion*

Quotation
You never get a second chance to make a first impression. – Author Unknown

Notation
Everyone receives a thought or feeling about someone or something upon observing, meeting or greeting. Sometimes this is based on little evidence, sometimes this view may change over time or it may remain the same. It is an opinion, view or judgement and its effects fleeting or long lasting.

Thrive on Five

1. Your being

When you choose something, you take aligned actions, not wish for something. Wishing, leaves you in a constant state of wishing for it. It is in the ether zone. When you act towards achieving your goal, each action accumulates to achieve success. Each action takes you in the direction you perceived, or in the direction of new opportunities to achieve your goal. People will see you as someone presenting yourself who wants your goal, and if they can, they will be enrolled in your journey and may even be able to help. It is who you are being that attracts people to you. It is the impression they perceive and the insights they gain from your being. Your energy.

2. Be yourself

How often have you heard a loved one, a teacher, or friend say this to you? Be yourself! Perhaps it is a new concept for you. Everyone, yes everyone has their own 'youniqueness.' Everyone has something to offer to their world and to the world. Observe from others you admire but remember to allow your gifts and talents to shine. What gifts and talents do you have that if channelled, could inspire, educate or create you a business or lifestyle you desire?

3. Take action

What is one action you could take today that would take you in the direction of living your dreams? Being in action shows to yourself, others and to the universe that you are committed to your dreams and goals. Make someday, one day, today! Live the life you love and love the life you live. Make that impression that reflects 'younique' you.

4. Trust your impressions

You may get a sense, a feeling, an idea, a thought or a hunch about something or someone. Trust this feeling. Your perception is usually correct and then you may second guess yourself and you find that you wished you trusted the initial feeling. Be guided by your own influence but remember it is your view, your opinion and your judgement from one viewpoint. Remember, everyone has their own viewpoint and that is why people have disagreeing perceptions about the same situation. Do you trust or act on first impressions?

5. Second chance

Whilst the quote by the unknown author says that first impressions are lasting, everyone is bigger than the biggest mistake they have made. Is there anyone you know who deserves a second chance? Of course, this does not mean placing yourself in harm's way and it does not mean you will forget any wrong doings, it is forgiveness of yourself and the other person. This could be done in person, or this could be done by releasing negative thoughts. This could also be done by personal development or with professional assistance. You will know what works for you.

Impress*ion* Summary

- Each aligned action, no matter how small, moves you in the direction of living your dreams.
- Trust your intuition.
- Be yourself. You are the only one who can be you.
- Forgive yourself for perceived wrongs.
- Forgiveness is a life-giving gift.

RAELENE DAL SANTO

5 views on knowledge and human connectedness

27. Information

Quotation
Knowledge is power. Information is liberating. Education is the premise of progress, in every society, in every family. – Kofi Annan

Notation
Information is enlightenment for yourself and others. It allows for learning and modifications. It allows for discussions which allows for solutions. Information allows access, it stimulates action, it helps with problem solving, and it helps us to be problem sensitive to fellow human beings.

Thrive on Five

1. Hope or fear

Corruption and subjugation occur when the knowledge of power is bound by no rules, no laws, no rights and no accountability. The universe is easily accessible and connected via information. The discerning and evaluation of such information is a skill, both with who provides it and how it is perceived. Information can engender hope, equally it can engender fear.

2. Information allows for emotions to be processed

Remember a time when you were scared and upset by not knowing something. Did it make you fearful and unable to proceed with clear thought processes, the ability to make a choice, or what to do next? More information, explained in a way that is meaningful to you allows for inner peace and calm, and when in this state, more informed choices can be made. Are you or someone you know dealing with something? Could information personally or professionally help you with the choice to enhance wellbeing. Who could you ask? What help would you like?

3. Reason for the season

There are more languages than the spoken and written languages of the world. There is the language of crafts, sports, music, gardening and whatever passion you are interested in. When you speak that language, it is another level of relate-ability to another human being. It sparks interest, dialogue and connectedness. Sometimes you meet strangers and they share information that impacts your life. Sometimes people in your life are there for short periods of time to share information and relatedness. Sometimes people are in your life forever and the connection is sometimes inexplicable and irreplaceable. Always remember in life, you are in the perfect place, time and space to learn information, until you are in another time and place to learn more information about your life journey.

4. Six degrees of separation (or as my brother says more like 1.6)

The digital information seems to link humanity in ways that seem explainable yet are inexplicable. Someone knows someone that knows someone. Remember with all this instant information, the following skills are important too: social skills, human interaction skills, life skills, citizenship skills and self-love skills. Be kind to yourself. Be kind to others. Information can help you to be 'mind-full.' Remember to be 'heart-full' too.

5. Information Industrial Revolution

Discovering your passion and what gives you access to information is empowering. With this, you can be, do and have what you want for your life. Creativity and productivity are words often spoken about when people are learning what brings fulfilment to their lives. When empowered and doing what they love, people are seemingly more joyous and sense success. The first Industrial Revolution saw production mechanised with the use of water and steam. The second Industrial Revolution allowed mass production using electric power. The third Industrial Revolution allows for electronics and information technology to automate production. As such, the world is now more closely linked with the access to information and the collaboration possible between people across it. How could your ideas use the automated information technology revolution?

Informat*ion* Summary

- Information allows access.
- Be problem solving.
- Be problem sensitive.
- Share hope.
- Information allows for relatability.

5 approaches to create with courage

28. Innovat*ion*

Quotation
Changes call for innovation, and innovation leads to progress. – Li Keqiang

Notation
Innovation requires change, transformation and restructure. Individuals, businesses, communities and countries are constantly creating newness, changing direction, and finding solutions to meet requirements current and perceived.

Innovate and create. Have courage, despite all the circumstances that may come forth. Remember a mighty and majestic oak tree grows from a tiny acorn. The seed needs nurturing, as does the tree. So, do you.

Thrive on Five

1. Begin somewhere

If you think you can, you are going to. If you think you can't, then most likely, you are not. Remember wherever you are in your stage of life, you need to begin somewhere and when you are somewhere, you begin again. You are renewing and creating at all ages and stages. Judge not, for what you have done, what you will do, and what you are doing, as they are all part of you. A characteristic of innovation is courage. Irish poet Oliver Goldsmith wrote, 'Success consists of getting up just one more time than you fall.' Have the courage to innovate your life, how you choose. Be courageous. Fall. Stand up. Trust and have faith. Create, innovate and enjoy your life.

2. Creative writing

What would you like to be, do or have? Quiet and calm your mind and allow yourself to be creative. Obviously, this could have a more scientific, complex, neuroscientific description of what occurs in the brain, but research shows that when we are calm, we make more measured choices. Choose an aspect of life, such as a hobby, sport, artistic, music or cultural pursuit that interests you. Think about this and write any thoughts, ideas, insights, messages and actions you receive. If you feel stuck, the act of writing allows ideas to flow and ideas to be out of your head. Writing can be releasing and revealing, helping to explore, create and innovate new possibilities.

3. Creating a partnership

Do you have a fabulous idea for business, leisure or your community? To allow this idea to be in the universe, do you need to form a partnership? For example, you produce organic meat or vegetables on your farm, but you need a retail outlet. You could create a partnership with a marketing agent to share your product with local consumers at markets or an online sale business. This could then mean you require refrigeration access for state or interstate deliveries. You do not need to do it all by yourself. A lesson everyone can learn and relearn. Connectedness is the key to good health and good business. Who could you connect with?

4. Play

The art of playing, being in the moment and creating games from what you have around you in the home, in the backyard, in your environment and in nature, allows you to be spontaneous and creative. Play is not just for children. Allow your inner child to be creative and joyous. Fun is an operative word for innovation.

5. Challenge yourself

Set yourself a challenge, a contest. Be it fitness, wellbeing, giving up something, or trying something new. Set a goal for a day, a week, a month, a year and write it down. What do you need to do, have and be to realise this challenge? Do you need to enrol the support of others? Commit time to do something for yourself each day. Find a way to find time for you.

Innovat*ion* Summary

- The oak tree acorn needs nurturing to be the mighty oak tree. So, do you.
- Writing or drawing allows you to see the visual picture, not just in the imagination.

LIVE WITH LOVE

- Innovate, create and communicate.
- Partnerships offer a different view.
- Be playful, have fun and remember the child within.

5 ideas for positive practice

29. Inspirat*ion*

Quotation
Stop being afraid of what could go wrong and think of what could go right.
– Yoana Dianika

Notation
The influence of a person, place or experience can allow you to think and feel in such a way that you want to be, do or have something in your life, or create something for the world. You could inspire someone by caring, acknowledging, listening, challenging, believing in and uplifting them. Be an example of integrity. To yourself. To others.

Thrive on Five

1. Who or what inspires you?
Who or what inspires you to be the best version of yourself? What stimulates creativity and how do you keep yourself inspired to achieve your goals and live a life you love? To invent, to innovate and to imagine are all results of inspiration. Jack Canfield said, 'Don't worry about failures, worry about the chances you miss when you don't even try.'

2. Feeling with the heart
Not all tangible things bring happiness. In terms of happiness, feelings of love and admiring beauty around and within are priceless. When someone is an inspiration, people admire and want to be like that. They want information and insights so that they too can see what is possible in the world and find what they need and want for themselves. What gives you inspiration? Inspiration can also come from observing, noticing and appreciating what surrounds your life. People, places, animals, sounds, colours, light, nature, smells and food can give you inspiration and ideas for both work and leisure pursuits.

3. Do the smallest acts
Every act adds up to success. Do what there is to do today, do your best, be in action and that is preparation for tomorrow, whilst living in the now. It is a reminder to be present. You notice this when you realise in the moment that you were over analysing things that have happened, or what may occur, neither which are happening now. Around you all the time are opportunities to perform random acts of kindness to people in your life, and in the world. These are free but are the most valued currency. Everyday random acts of kindness include

smiling, being courteous, using manners, saying something kind, sometimes saying nothing at all, asking someone if they are okay, and having integrity. Commit to what you said you would do, by when you said you would. What is a random act of kindness you could do today?

4. Let go of that which no longer serves
Not all plans go as we choose or want, whether it is a dream, a plan, an action or a desire. Finding a way to grieve it and to forgive yourself, is a way to live the life that is now awaiting you. Do what is in front of you and what is possible, and you will see that new possibilities arise. New opportunities will be around and so will people, to offer a kind word or an idea. This is the same of things, people, jobs, dreams and goals. If it no longer serves you or what you are up to in life, then perhaps it is a time to release and let go? This may not be easy. It takes strength and courage and it also takes kindness and compassion for yourself.

5. Be someone's rainbow
Sometimes for whatever reason, someone needs support. Being there for someone is an act of kindness. Maya Angelou suggests we could, 'Try to be a rainbow in someone's cloud.' Sometimes a hug, a smile, a kind word, even no words at times, are the most valuable gifts. How could you be a rainbow for someone? Choose a colour you love and shine it brightly. This is your moment to inspire.

Inspirat*io*n Summary
- Who or what inspires you to be the best version of you?
- You will have a relationship with you your whole life.

LIVE WITH LOVE

- Love is priceless.
- Today is a good day to live your dream and let go of what does not serve you anymore.
- Every aligned action adds up to success.

5 ideas to be right here and right now

30. Location

Quotation
There is a plan and a purpose, a value to every life, no matter what its location, age, gender or disability. – Sharron Angle

Notation
Location, in this book, is a reference of where you are physically and or emotionally. So, it can be a geographical or external place where you live, work or study, or an internal, social emotional setting within.

Thrive on Five

1. Where are you now?

Wherever we are in life, it provides lessons. Would you like to live somewhere else? Why? Could you achieve this feeling of where you would like to live, temporarily where you are now? For example, if you love the ocean, but you live in the city, you could decorate your home with pictures, furniture or accessories that remind you of the ocean. You could plan a weekend getaway to the ocean with family and friends. You could take up a hobby involving the ocean. You could train or retrain for an occupation involving the ocean. Plan. Create. Enjoy.

2. Vision board

Use photos, pictures, or create artwork to decorate your home or workplace of places you love to be or would love to be. Create digital vision boards, which can be easily accessible as a screensaver, visible whenever you access your device. A visual representation is a reminder to your mind and heart what you would like in the physical world.

3. Declutter

Declutter your home to create a more loving energetic space. Decluttering can remove negative energy and allow space for positive energy. It can rejuvenate the soul and feel like you have been on a vacation. Removing the weight of physical possessions, allows for the associated emotional load to be lifted from your environment and energy field. This book may help you declutter, *The Life Changing Magic of Tidying Up: The Japanese Art of Decluttering and Organising*, by Marie Kondo.

4. Plan a holiday

Plan a local, national or international holiday. Holidays are your design, from budget to luxurious, home or abroad, adventurous or relaxing, and alone or with others. Design your own holiday or discuss your needs with a professional travel agent. Plan it. Live it. Love it.

5. Visit family and friends
If you are looking for an inexpensive yet uplifting and connecting holiday, you could stay with those you know. Visit loved ones and get away from your own surrounds. A physical break can be an emotional break. It provides connections in a real, not just a digital way. Who could you connect with?

Locat*ion* Summary

- You are right here, right now. Begin here.
- Allow yourself to dream.
- Does your current location suit your needs and wants?
- Release thoughts and things that no longer serve you.
- To recharge, do you need a homestay or getaway?

5 nurturing and restorative ways of being

31. Meditat*ion*

Quotation
Sleep is the best meditation. – Dalai Lama

Notation
The benefits of meditation are being researched to help reduce stress, anxiety, upset and pain. Meditation is like art, nothing is wrong, nothing is right. It is personal interpretation. Find a way that works for you.

Thrive on Five

1. Breath control or just breathe

Breath control is something you can try almost anywhere. Breathe deeply and exhale slowly. Focus on what makes you calm. Have pictures of people and places near you that bring you joy. Play calming music and create calm spaces. Research meditation and perhaps find a group near you. Find a book, class or teacher and learn a way that works for you.

2. Find time for you

Initially find 10 minutes a day to be still, calm and present. In this moment breathe and learn, breathe and listen, breathe and be. There is nothing to do, nowhere to go, no one to be. Just be you. Just be.

3. Exercise and or stretch

Whatever activity and level of intensity you choose to do, depends on your own personal needs and your daily energy. Remember to move, as exercise can also give you energy. Exercise can improve strength, stiffness, cardiovascular fitness, sleep and general physical function. Seek medical or health advice if unsure of your needs and capabilities.

4. Sleep rests the body and mind

Sleep is essential for life. The restorative power of sleep assists optimal daily function. It is vital to wellbeing and health. Research good sleep habits to see if you could improve your sleep patterns, sleep environments, sleep routines and sleep length. Seek medical or health care advice if sleep is of concern to your wellbeing.

5. Yoga, Tai Chi and Qi Gong

These are all meditative forms of exercise, with postures and breath control, that keep you present. When you perform an exercise, stretch or movement you are more focused, therefore not being distracted by things occurring in your life. These activities provide physical, emotional and social benefits, contributing to your wellbeing.

Meditation Summary

- Breathe. Connect with your breath.
- Inhale love, exhale fear.
- Be calm and present.
- Restorative sleep is a key to good health.
- Movement gives you energy. Find a type of movement that works for you.

5 ways to create a vision and venture to achieve it

32. Mot*ion*

Quotation
If you can't fly then run, if you can't run then walk, if you can't walk then crawl, but whatever you do you have to keep moving forward. – Martin Luther King Jnr

Notation
The famous words of Martin Luther King Jnr were to inspire his audience to keep moving in the direction of their dreams, despite objects both perceived and physical that may be along the path of life. He encouraged people to push beyond their limits and to have no limitations.

Thrive on Five

1. Nature in motion
Nature is in constant motion with the ebbs and flows of the tides, the cycles of life, the constant change, and the transformation of one way to another. Nature has its own rhythmical dance and it creates the music. Humans too have continual and ever changing needs and wants. This is human emotion in motion. Motion occurs within and around you.

2. Vision then venture
Hold onto your dream and with each action along your journey, you will achieve. Life after all, is a series of journeys. How often do you see people you know or people in the media creating and recreating, and sharing something current in alignment with their dreams? Dreams evolve and may change. Dreams may be many. It is like Sebastian Terry, Founder of *100 Things* and *Kindsum* suggests, once something is achieved on the 'What's on your list?' it is onto the next venture. Be in motion. Be in action. Enjoy the journey of your dreams. Enjoy sharing others dreams. Enjoy your day.

3. You've got to move it
You may have heard the phrase 'move it' and medical experts advocate it. Being physically fit is not a place to be, it is a way to be. Like life, there is no destination, it is a journey. It is a continual process of motion. Motion for the body, is also motivation for the mind and satisfaction for the soul. What is one change you could do and be today, for a healthier you?

4. Wandering

You may feel you wander, seemingly without direction but it is motion, nonetheless. It is moving, not being stationary. At times, it may feel like you do not know your direction, but you are on a carefree wander of discovery, or perhaps a wander with a destination in mind. A wander is a wander, still in motion. Sometimes when you do this you create situations and opportunities arise, that you did not know were possible. Sometimes a wander can be time out from life's seeming monotony. Sometimes it is motion in a different direction. Do you need to stop wandering or begin it? Motion towards what you want for your life.

5. Information to motion

If information is knowledge, and knowledge is power, to make a difference in your life or in the life of someone else, what prevents you from putting your intention into motion? Why do you know that exercise is vital for health and not be in motion? Why do you know that food with nutritional value is better than foods without and yet you make an unhealthy choice? Only two examples but knowing and doing, are two very different things. What is the key for action? What is the key that would allow your life to be in motion? What is an action you could take today to make your health, hobby, interest, study, work, family or personal goals and dreams a reality, not just a dream? Who would you need to be, to be in motion, resulting in effective action?

Mot*ion* Summary

- Dream your vision and venture with action.
- Move it. Just keep moving.

- Take time out to be and be with your creative thoughts.
- Learning is knowledge and knowledge is power.
- Be in motion and action to achieve your goals and dreams.

5 inspiring ways to action your goals and dreams

33. Motivat*ion*

Quotation
The only impossible journey is the one you never begin. – Tony Robbins

Notation
Eleanor Roosevelt said, 'The future belongs to those who believe in the beauty of their dreams.' Sometimes in the quest to achieve your goals and dreams the road requires navigation of your own doubts, the critical analysis of others and obstacles perceived and real. At times the doubt may seem more powerful than the goal and it may seem unattainable. What motivates your own resolution to succeed?

Thrive on Five

1. What is your dream?
'If you can dream it, you can do it,' said Walt Disney. Find a way to fulfil your dream, to leave your legacy in the world, but most importantly so you live a fulfilled life you love, with love. Be real with you. What is it that gives your life sparkle and joy? What are your dreams? In realising your dream there may be obstacles, doubters, self-doubt, lessons and lots of effort. But similarly, there will be strength of mind, courage of heart and success. Live your dreams.

2. You will find a way
Remember to trust yourself, back yourself and find a way. This may come in many forms. Be open and aware to notice the signs of assistance on the journey, be it a word, a saying, a person, an invitation or an insight. There are people who may criticise and be jealous but there are many more who will be constructive, joyous and helpful. Share your dreams and any assistance you need as you will find others willing and able to help along the road of kindness. Another reminder of finding a way is by Harriet Beecher Stowe, 'Never give up, for that is just the place and the time that the tide will turn.'

3. Motivation vs Procrastination
Procrastination is the distraction from dream fulfilment. The 'what ifs,' the 'I cant's,' the 'oh I have to,' and all similar thought or spoken excuses, distracting you from your purpose and passions. The little killjoys of your own doubts or other opinions, block and stop you. What are your distraction words and actions? What have you stopped yourself from being, doing or having? What dream is left unfulfilled inside of you, that

procrastination has you at the orange traffic light of life? What is one action you could do for yourself today that would move you towards your dream? Remember the words of Theodore Roosevelt, 'Keep your eyes on the stars, and your feet on the ground.'

4. Start somewhere. Begin the Journey. Enjoy your journey.

Tennis great Arthur Ashe said, 'To achieve greatness, start where you are, use what you have, do what you can.' Be inspired by others. Use their motivation and courage to help you step towards your dream. Listen to the voices of the people that inspire you to be the best version of yourself. Listen to those who believe in you and your dreams, to those who hear that your contribution to the world matters, and to those that can see you bigger than you can see yourself. Most importantly, listen to 'younique' you.

5. Manifestation of the right person or circumstance, at the right time

Share your dreams and what is going on for you. Sharing allows you to find the people and the resources you may need to execute your dreams. In my life, each setback, each quote, each journal note, each observation of nature and humanity, each action, each heartache and each moment motivated me and contributed to this book. Following motivation from other authors, support from family and friends and the commitment to myself and my dream is what mattered. What is your commitment to yourself? Sam Levenson said, 'Don't watch the clock, do what it does. Keep going.'

Motivat*ion* Summary

- Identify your goal and dreams. What is it you want to be, do and have?
- Believe in yourself and your dreams.
- Follow your heart.
- Share your goals and dreams and notice the people and opportunities that cross your path.
- Listen and learn from others but listen and learn from yourself too.

5 ways food sustains life

34. Nutrit*ion*

Quotation
Our food should be our medicine and our medicine should be our food. – Hippocrates

Notation
Natures gift of food guides humans to eat by the seasons. Listen you your own inner wisdom. Learn from the wisdom of the universe. The nature of the food you eat depends on your personal situation including location and accessibility to food, national and international regulations and the types of foods you can eat for your stage of development and any health conditions.

Jamie Oliver is one of my favourite chefs. His aim and his passion are summarised in the quote, 'What I've enjoyed most, though, is meeting people who have a real interest in food and sharing ideas with them. Good food is a global issue and I find that there is always something new and amazing to learn – I love it!' This is evident in his passion not only for food and nutrition, but for family, friends and human connectedness.

Thrive on Five

1. Family models

Nutrition is the absorbing of nutrients from foods, in relation to the body's needs. Study and learn about foods that are for you, as a well human being. My Grandma passed away in 2012, aged 98, from old age. If she didn't know what it was or who made it, she did not eat it. Hot water was the first thing she drank, believing it aided digestion, followed by food half an hour later. This was for everything she ate, every meal time, every day. Whilst this is only one thing she did for her wellbeing, she did it. Grandad and Grandma grew their own vegetables. She didn't drive and used to walk ten kilometres a day. She was conscious that chemicals did not enter her body, via hair, skin or ingestion. She was conscious and present to the needs of her body. Particular? Yes. Admirable? Yes. Jack LaLanne's quote is apt here for Grandma, 'Exercise is King, Nutrition is Queen. Put them together and you've got a Kingdom.' Do you have people in your life who model good nutrition practices?

2. Your health

Ralph Waldo Emerson said, 'The first wealth is health.' What to eat is individual. If you have any health queries seek your inner wisdom and medical assistance or advice. Experts in their field can offer suggestions to improve health and wellbeing. Nutrition to humans is power to function, just like fuel or a power source help a vehicle to function. Understanding your body's individual needs and how it works is essential to optimum functioning. How are you feeling? Is there anything you need to do or to let go of? Do you need to have a check up with a medical or health care provider?

3. Seasonal produce

Grow seasonal produce in your home, garden or in a community garden. Read about gardening, complete a gardening course, ask your local nursery for advice, watch lifestyle programs, join a gardening group and make connections. Agricultural methods allow some foods to be grown all year. Nature shares what is grown by the seasons. Dad is my family supplier of fresh seasonal produce. Very grateful.

4. Buy bulk for your family or as a group

Collectively bulk buy fresh fruit and vegetables with family, friends or neighbours. Obviously, this depends on where you live and involves planning meals, food preferences, and catering for any individual health needs or dietary requirements. You could buy fresh food from supermarkets, co-operatives or seek out country, coastal, city or grower's markets.

5. Growers' market

Find a local growers' market connecting farmers direct to consumers in your area. Discover farmers online who send you food boxes direct. Learn about the variety of regional, national and international foods. Create communities where local artisans and growers sell their goods and provide a service. If one does not exist in your area, perhaps this is an opportunity for you to create access for yourself and others. Eating in local cafes and restaurants that utilise local produce is also a way of appreciating farmers and the food service industry of your area. You could make a family favourite recipe or create your own.

Nutrition Summary

- Choose seasonal produce if available.

- Nutrition is important for optimal health.
- Understand your body and its nutritional needs.
- Food sustains life.
- The provision of food is a personal, national and global issue.

5 ways to notice the beauty of life

35. Observation

Quotation
The power of accurate observation is commonly called cynicism by those who have not got it. – George Bernard Shaw

Notation
Be still and be an observer of your thoughts and feelings for your own wellbeing and healing. Energy moves around and within you all the time. Be calm and allow energy to move gently around your body and be a silent observer of this movement. Self-awareness, self-regulation and self-realisation comes from profound self-observation.

Thrive on Five
1. Meditation
Meditation is an *'ion'* word covered in the book, so for here I will just write, breathe. Calm, close your eyes, breathe and allow your thoughts to come and let them go, like waves rolling onto shore and back out. Breathe. If it is not your thing to sit and close your eyes, then sit somewhere peaceful and quiet, or imagine you are at your favourite place. Just breathe. Yes, it's involuntary for the respiratory system of the body to do this for you, but how you breathe can be a conscious choice. Breathe and breathe slowly. Breath control compliments calmness for the mind and may assist with self-regulation.

2. Notice children being present
Here I am referring to the mindful moments of being present in the now. Remember to when you were a child. What is a special memory of childhood? Who had a profound influence upon or was an inspiration to you? What goals and dreams did you have for yourself? What is one child like thing you could do to make yourself laugh and bring joy to your life. Perhaps jump in puddles, kick a pile of leaves, make a snow angel or roll down a hill. What brings you joy? If this seems self-absorbed or self-centred, recreate these moments as self-discovery, self-perception and self-fulfilment. A lot of self-analysis can be learned by observing children play and being present.

3. Observe others
Watch, learn and acquire knowledge and wisdom by observing. Watch how others handle situations, how they speak, what words they use and their nature. By observing, you can then process your thoughts and work out what works for you, what

plans and ideas you would like to implement for you and your lifestyle. Observing gives you an opportunity to be, rather than do. Observe the actions that speak louder than words.

4. Observe nature

Nature has a way of teaching you about the cycle and lessons of life, some of it brutal and some of it beautiful. Nature has a powerful way of grounding you to Mother Earth and its nurturing effects on the body, mind and soul. As I write, I am sitting at a café near the ocean. The sun is streaming down warm rays, the smell of salt is in the air, the gentle waves roll in, the sky is blue with some scattered clouds, and I can hear fellow *caferians* (do you like my word?) chatter and natter. There are even a few people practicing salsa dancing on the footpath. It is a stimulus of the senses and yet here I can focus and write. It is a place that gives me inspiration and rejuvenates my soul, and the coffee is fabulous. Where is your favourite spot to observe nature and humanity? Be it home, mountains, rivers, lakes, oceans, rainforests, parks, desert, farmlands, savanna or wetlands.

5. Sensibility

Your senses are continually observing, interpreting, classifying and making sense of information from your surrounds and within. The nature of your observation of the external world can impact your physiological functioning and your interactions with the world. Remember each person observes the world differently and each person can make different observances, even of the same observation.

Observat*ion* Summary

LIVE WITH LOVE

- Self-observation is a gift.
- Be aware of the messages of your own reflection.
- Breathe. Calm the mind and body. This helps self-regulation.
- Wisdom comes from observation of self and others.
- Observe the rhythms of nature. Be in nature.

5 ways to embrace life with grace

36. Opin*ion*

Quotation
Everyone is entitled to his own opinion, but not his own facts. – Daniel Patrick Moynihan

Notation
Your view or judgement about someone or something is an opinion. It may be based on fact or knowledge or not. Remember human essence is behind that stereotype or view. Is it a view of fear or a view of love? It is an opinion.

Thrive on Five

1. Does it really matter?

In the book *The Alchemist*, Paolo Coelho said, 'If someone isn't what others want them to be, the others become angry. Everyone seems to have a clear idea of how other people should lead their lives, but none about his or her own.' Everyone has an opinion. No one's is more important than another. Everyone is entitled to their opinion. Do you have to like it? No. Do you have to follow it? No. Doesn't mean you like it, follow it, endorse it, want it, need it, value it, or think it serves a higher good for yourself or others. It is an opinion. Surprisingly, you may learn something, when an opinion seems diametrically opposed to your opinion. Find the lesson, Be grateful for the lesson. You cannot change others, just the way you view your world, and the world.

2. Everyone is entitled to their own opinion

Why is that? Why is everyone entitled to their opinion? Asking someone why they think something, can give you an insight into their understanding and perspective on a topic. When you actively listen, and learn, it creates for a more enjoyable interaction than dismissing their opinion. But be aware, some people may interpret the opinion quotation as, 'Everyone is entitled to their opinion.' Perhaps a narcissistic view shrouded in either fear or arrogance, or both. Listen and learn. Life and people always give you an opportunity to learn. To learn what you want, as well as what you do not want, for yourself or your life.

3. Do you have an opinion?

In *The Diary of a Young Girl*, Anne Frank said, 'People can tell you to keep your mouth shut, but that doesn't stop you from having your own opinion.' Your opinion matters. Silence can keep you safe, speaking can set you free. Not only to you, but it may contribute to enhance the lives of others. If safe, speak up. Your voice is valid. Be powerful. Share the 'younique' you the world needs. Be in communication and collaboration with others. Share your gifts, talents, skills, knowledge and words with your world, and the world. Use your voice to speak up and someone will be there to listen.

4. What people think of you

Mum taught me, 'What other people think of you, is none of your business.' Meaning that what you think of you and those whose opinion matter to you, is what matters. Respect other people's opinion. Respect your opinion. In both cases ask these questions. Is it truth? Is it fact? Is it proven? Perhaps yes, perhaps no. It is their opinion. Is it for you? Listen to your inner wisdom and guidance. Try something, if it works, great. If not, learn from it and with different information, try something else.

5. Be a voice for those who do not feel they have a voice that is heard

Who or what would benefit from your voice? Be it for an individual, community group or an organisation, someone needs your voice. Remember one voice can be louder than a noisy crowd. One voice can lead. Let Nelson Mandela's following words remind you of this, 'I learned that courage was not the absence of fear, but the triumph over it. The brave man is not he who does not feel afraid, but he who conquers that fear.' For who or what do you need to use your voice? When he visited Australia in 2000, I was privileged and humbled to listen to the wisdom and forgiveness of Nelson Mandela.

Opin*ion* Summary

- What are your values?
- You are entitled to an opinion. Everyone is.
- Listen and learn even when someone's opinion seems diametrically opposed to yours?
- Release thoughts and things that no longer serve you.
- Be a voice for those who may not have the opportunity to speak or be heard.

5 compassionate ways to make a difference

37. Organisation

Quotation
Three rules of work: Out of clutter find simplicity. From discord find harmony. In the middle of difficulty lies opportunity. – Albert Einstein

Notation
In this context of organisation, I am referring to planning, coordinating and being responsible for yourself, your belongings, and at times for others. Organisation of thoughts, yourself, others and your environment, help you choose what will be your next action.

Thrive on Five

1. Disorganisation to organisation

Finding places for things, and putting things in places, may bring peace and calm to the cluttered mind. Organisation is being able to sort what was, what is, what is yet to come, and what you will do with the evaluation of this information. Leonardo Da Vinci said, 'Simplicity is the ultimate sophistication.' Do you need help from disorganisation to organisation? What requires organisation in your life? Who could you ask for help?

2. Organisation of thoughts

Thoughts constantly come and go through the mind. Living and loving the life you live, is learning to decipher which thoughts to give your attention to and which to let go. Napoleon Hill describes this in the quote, 'First comes thought, then organisation of that thought, into ideas and plans: then transformation of those plans into reality. The beginning, as you will observe, is in your imagination.'

3. Self-organisation

It is necessary to regulate and organise yourself so that you can function to achieve the actions of your endeavours. How you organise yourself is personal to your life and lifestyle. Whether you function in a creative mess, tidy idleness or a mixture of both, is up to you. If what you are doing is working and achieving results then great. If not, then seek assistance to organise your belongings, ideas or time, so that you can function efficiently to achieve the results you choose or are required of you.

4. Organisation of and for others

Whether within your family, home, learning or work environment, the organisation and team effort required as well as the accomplishments are a combined result of each person. You may be in a caring, supportive or leadership role, either voluntary or paid, but the elements of management and contribution are similar. These positions require you to inspire, educate, inform, communicate and lead. In each situation, there is commitment, trust and integrity. When people feel valued, they become happier and more successful. Being grateful for someone's contribution no matter how small, contributes to the overall function of a team. Saying a genuine thank you is much appreciated.

5. Organisation of your environment

This could be of the surrounding material and physical possessions, or the relationships within your environment. Weaving the tapestry of relationships is an unwritten, unchartered area. There may be rules and regulations, but human nature is like the ever-changing unchartered depths of the ocean. It is the informal organisation within formal organisations. Details need attention. Priorities help with productivity. Do you need assistance organising the physical or human resources in your environment?

Organisation Summary

- Where in your life do you inspire, educate, inform, communicate and lead?
- Organising your thoughts helps to organise your life.
- How do you organise the physical and human resources

in your environment?
- Release thoughts and things that no longer serve you.
- Structures help with organisation and when it has served the purpose, re organise the structure.

5 ideas to discover and live your dreams

38. Pass*ion*

Quotation

My mission in life is not merely to survive, but to thrive and to do so with some passion, some compassion, some humour and some style. – Maya Angelou

Notation

Passion as referred to in this book, is the enthusiasm, energy, commitment and excitement for someone or something. A person's eagerness or intensity for something can be contagious. Remember a time you met someone and their energy for what they do and who they are being, elevated you to follow your dream. Their exuberance is exciting, their happiness is heart-warming. Passion can often drive social, political, financial, health, wellbeing, and emotional choices and for an individual, a cause, a community or an organisation. What are you passionate about?

Thrive on Five

1. What is your passion?

What is your passion? What gives sparkle and adds magic to your life? What would you choose to do, have or be, for paid or even unpaid work? Is it a profession, sport, an art, music, job, social pursuit, lifestyle, community affiliation or a social cause? What do you need to discover and follow for this passion? If you are unsure, a great book for guidance already mentioned is *What Colour is Your Parachute?* by Richard N Bolles.

2. Follow your passion

Are you in a vocation, relationship, lifestyle or location that allows you to be who you would like to be? Do you have the resources so you can live your life with passion, following your passion? Are there any changes you need to make to fulfil your purpose and passion in life? Only you will know the answer to these questions.

3. Be honest with yourself

Read the following question and honestly answer without self-judgement, doubt or questioning. An honest answer will come and what you do with that inner answer is up to you. Life takes you in all different directions and this could just be in the same day. Be, do and have what you would like and allow your light to shine into your world. Here is the question. If time, money and all the resources you needed were infinite, what would you like to be, do or have in this world? Answer quickly, without hesitation, or evaluation of what answer comes to you. Journal all the ideas that arise. Write and write. Then read. Are there any clues for you to take the next step towards your dream? What resources both physical and financial or personal do you need?

Live your dream. Live your life. *Live with Love*. Create with love. Enjoy with love.

4. Guidance
Louise Hay shares in her book, *The Power is Within You*, that you have the resources within to achieve your goals and that you are stronger than you know yourself to be. Meditation allows for connection to self. Breathing calmly and connecting to your inner voice provides guidance. When the noise of the outside world is quiet, you can connect to your inside world and the infinity of the universe.

5. Guidance from others
Others may offer and be open to guidance. It is a gift, as it allows family, friends, colleagues and even strangers to contribute to your life. Listen and learn. The words someone speaks may just give you the spark, the idea, the resource, the tool, or the energy to bring forth your passion into the world, for you and for service to others. Ask for guidance, seek guidance and follow your own guidance.

Pass*ion* Summary
- What or who brings joy to your life?
- What brings sparkle to your life?
- Is there some creative passion or adventure yearning within that needs to be in existence?
- Ask for guidance where required? It allows others to contribute to your life.
- Be honest with yourself. Are you living a life you love?

5 ways to conceive, believe and achieve

39. Preparat*ion*

Quotation
Prior preparation prevents poor performance. – James Baker

Notation
The Greek Philosopher Aristotle said, 'We are what we repeatedly do. Excellence, then, is not an act, but a habit.' This applies to the time and effort spent on positive aspects that enhance our lives as well as the negative habits we have that we may be conscious or not conscious of. This is regarding people and such things as places, foods, drinks, words and jobs. You will put up with things for whatever reason, until you make a conscious choice to move away, let go and release that which holds you back, or has you in a holding pattern, like the orange traffic light flashing at you. You need to proceed and get the green light.

Thrive on Five

1. Preparation is key

Preparation is the passion and commitment to something in the short term, for a long-term gain. It is about goals, determination, planning and actioning the plan. Realise it is small steps to mastery, like learning that the marathon finishes at the end, and the race is part of that, step by step. Whilst not everyone is a marathon runner, it is learning that to achieve your goal and contribute your 'younique' skills and talents to the world, it requires planning and commitment. First the commitment is to yourself and then for others. Acknowledge your steps to mastery.

2. Choose an aspect of your life

Choose an area of your life you would like to improve or develop. Research and read about the topic you are interested in. What skills or resources do you need? Who could you ask to assist you? Are there courses in your local area or online? Do you need a mentor, coach or personal trainer? How can you keep yourself accountable to attain your goal when you feel like quitting or have self-doubts? Intention followed by action is the preparation key.

3. What are you prepared to put up with and not?

Do you have what is required so that you are prepared for personal or professional pursuits? Are you needing to commit more time and energy to a project, work, study, person or even yourself? Find ten minutes a day to ponder, dream, focus, plan or take time out for you. Create time intervals of ten minutes to do something for yourself. Take ten minutes of time to sit, relax, and write down all your creative ideas or gratitude thoughts for the day. Take ten minutes to sit or walk in nature and feel its relaxing, calming effects. Even ten minutes can seem like a long time.

4. Do you need a coach, mentor or personal trainer?
Do you think or feel that you need to achieve and be everything on your own? Allowing others to contribute to your life, allows you to receive and them to give. The energy balance of giving and receiving is a gift for everyone to learn. Allowing others to contribute is a positive not a negative. It allows for connection and the collaboration of ideas that may not have been created. Love, intimacy and human connection is much needed in the world.

5. Team preparation
Teams have objectives and the individuals within may need preparation both personal and professional, to cohesively work together. Leading by example, sharing progress achievements, respecting each member, gratitude for accomplishments, being sensitive, positive and having fun are some practices that may help create such cohesion. What aspect of your life requires you to be a leader or leader of a team?

Preparat*ion* Summary
- Identify and commit to your passion.
- Complete daily actions toward your goal.
- Allow others to contribute to your life.
- Giving and receiving are life lessons of energy exchange.
- Connectedness is a human need.

5 ways of providing a sanctuary for self, others, nature and ideas

40. Protect*ion*

Quotation
I've learned that people will forget what you said, people will forget what you did, but people will never forget how you made them feel. – Maya Angelou

Notation
Safeguarding your sanctuary of self, your security wherever you are and the safety of loved ones, is paramount. Protection is an overarching human need and extends beyond the personal, to national and international, constitutional, economic and civil protections. Protection of self, being protected by others or the protection by something, provides sanctuary and security. This could be a feeling, a state of being, a physical presence or a physical building. Whatever provides shelter to your sense of protection is your protection. The sense of being safe is personal, and whilst constitutional protections both civil and political exist for some people, this is not so for all global citizens. Who, what, where and how do you feel protected?

Thrive on Five

1. Self-protection

Protection of yourself and your wellbeing is paramount. This includes physical, emotional, mental, and social wellbeing. Self-defence is a form of physical and mental security. Humans seek security and assurance for many things in life. This includes work or an income supply, health and wellbeing, home comfort and shelter from nature, and a sense of stability and civil security. As much as one seeks and deserves this most basic human right, not everyone is afforded this privilege. Too often security is taken for granted, until it is not present. Who or what gives you gratitude for personal security?

2. The feeling of protection

The feeling of comfort and safety that a home or shelter gives, is mental as well as physical comfort and wellbeing. The feeling of security and freedom is not to be underestimated. Think of a time you felt threatened or distressed and remember what calmed you, what made you feel safe and secure. What provided that inner feeling that everything will be okay? Again, not everyone is afforded this comfort, this access to physical and mental ease, this solace, help and support. The convenience some take for granted is a dream for others.

3. Possessions of protection

What possessions of comfort and ease of lifestyle could you donate, so that others would be afforded some basic comforts for restorative sleep, comfortable clothing and home comforts? What is in excess in your home that would help create a home or home feeling for another? Could you donate your time to a charity or organisation to assist others?

4. Protection of others

In some places, governments and individuals have strongholds over others by intimidation or threat, bribery, payoffs, extortion, remuneration, blackmail, gratuity, blocking of resources, exactions and corruption. People around the world use their position, power and influence to fight for their own civil rights and for those of others. This helps to provide support for others to help access the liberties, resources, support, and protection for both personal and home security. Sometimes you need to stand up for that which has been knocked down or taken away. Within regulatory limits, how could you help yourself, someone else or an organisation, feel supported and protected?

5. Building protection

Safety and protection from the elements of nature, and as a refuge, is provided by buildings or structures. The types of material used in construction of the protective covering, access to basic provisions of water, power supply and sanitation vary. Many do not have a fortified dwelling, a stronghold on their home, or any means to access anything different. This could result from personal, geographical or political reasons and restrictions. Governments and foreign aid aim to supply this most basic human need for shelter and safety, as well as the protection and safeguard of food and water supplies. How do you safeguard your own building protection? How could you assist the protection of someone else's basic needs of survival?

Protect*ion* Summary

- Where, what or who is your sanctuary, giving you the feeling of being safe and protected?

- Self-protection is paramount to wellbeing.
- Not everyone is afforded the feeling of protection.
- What place in the world do you feel most comfortable or at home?
- Where does your heart feel happy?

5 ways life mirrors a message to you

41. Reflect*ion*

Quotation

Without deep reflection one knows from daily life that one exists for other people. – Albert Einstein

Notation

Famous words by James Dean are, 'Dream as if you'll live forever, live as if you'll die today.' His quote and subsequent short life are both a cause and a pause for reflection. Tony Robbins quote also reminds us that, 'Setting a goal is the first step in turning the invisible into the visible.' Reflect on your goals. What is one step you could do today, that would move you one step towards achieving your goal or dream? It is like this quote by an unknown author, 'If we all don't row, the boat won't go.'

Thrive on Five

1. Universal alignment
The universe (or whatever word you would like to use) seems to align once we act and do the next action. The late Louise Hay, author, philanthropist and businesswoman was a renowned pioneer of positive affirmations of thinking and speaking. I was privileged to attend a course in Sydney, Australia at which she presented. When asked how her company became the successful Hay House, she said she did what was in front of her. Then she did the next thing and the next. How will reflection lead you to take a step closer to your goal or dream?

2. Rear view mirror reflection
Whilst it is important to be in the present and plan things for the future, it is good to self-reflect on where you have come from and then see how far you have progressed and keep progressing. Acknowledge yourself for your accomplishments. You learn by tweaking and making modifications and again keep going. Just like the Wright brothers did. They adjusted past flight performances and continued to trial and implement their ideas until they had success.

3. Reflection combination
Observation allows for the collection of information via acquisition of knowledge and by the senses. Reflection combines both and allows you to apply this to suit your life and lifestyle. Reflection can bring strength and courage and allows a view which may not have been apparent without it. Resolution is a result of reflection. Hence the making of them on the reflection of year's end leads to a new beginning of being better. Application is the key that helps you gain further knowledge

and observation. Appreciation and gratitude create more abundance. Reflection, observation, collection, information, acquisition, resolution, application, appreciation, and then reflection again. Notice all the *'ion'* words. It all starts over and is also intertwined. This, like life, is a continual cycle and journey. What do you need to release or to commence?

4. Mirror. Mirror.
The mirror image of you is not the total image. Consider the view of loved ones and ask how you occur for them in the world. Ask them to give you their feelings about your strengths and perceived weaknesses, bearing in mind that one could also be the other. Listen to the opinions of those that matter to you but always listen to your own inner voice. You are more than the image; you are also the inner refection of the words you speak and the character you are. Be kind to yourself and be reflective to open new windows to your inner mind.

5. Life reflection
Do you have a job, hobby or interest that reflects your life, both how it is and how you would like it to be? In that, you set a goal and you work out all the actions required to achieve this. Your life activity and attitude will reflect this both mentally and physically. Your life will have challenges, but you will also have triumphs. What reflects your life? How is it journaled or shared with the world? How does it reflect the emotions of your life journey? How do you express your creativity and experiences of life in the world?

Reflect*ion* Summary

- Be present, but at times remember where you came from

and where you want to go.
- Be proud of your accomplishments and remember the small steps to mastery.
- Learn from both perceived rights and wrongs.
- Take in the universe using all your senses.
- Life is a precious gem and over time it becomes more valuable.

5 guiding ways to regenerate your spirit

42. Rejuvenat*ion*

Quotation
Spring is nature's way of saying, 'Let's party!' – Robin Williams

Notation
Each day of each season has a lesson for you. Listen to your inner voice and it will guide you to what you need and want. Be kind to yourself and have patience with yourself. Renewing, rejuvenating and regeneration is a process. Ralph Waldo Emerson, said, 'Adopt the pace of nature; her secret is patience.' Be kind to yourself. Be kind to those you know, those you love and those you don't know. Everyone is trying the best they can. Be gracious with yourself. Be grateful for the kind deeds of others. Notice the world around you. Little things can rejuvenate your faith, your spirit, your soul.

Thrive on Five

1. The cycle of nature
Wake up and be outside in the natural light and enjoy the newness of sunrise. Similarly, if you are an evening person, enjoy the sunset. There is calmness in the rhythm of nature with its rejuvenating cycles of beginning and ending, of invigorating and regenerating. The cycles of nature will show you to be grateful for what was, what is, and to welcome what will be.

2. Foodalicious
Create a menu, bake or cook. Eat your favourite foods by yourself or with family and friends. Being with people you love is rejuvenating for the soul. Laughter, fun and good times are like a mini-vacation. I love how food brings people together to celebrate and create or to remember happy and special times. Rejoice in the memories that connecting and being with others brings. What are your favourite family recipes?

3. Press refresh
Try something new to revive, enliven and refresh yourself. Stop. Press pause. Sit. Be calm. Count to ten. Take three deep breaths. Could you approach something in a different way? Does the task need to be done right now? Who could you ask for help? What could you do just for you? Stop. Pause. Go.

4. Move it. Move it.
Set yourself a physical goal and write actions to achieve this. Depending on your connotation, the word exercise conjures up pleasant and/or unpleasant thoughts. Find an activity that you feel is fun and incorporate this with movement. You could catch up with a friend but instead of sitting down talking, you

could walk and talk. Share your health goal with trusted family and friends so they can help keep you accountable to realise your goals. Action rejuvenation, by choosing what works for you and your lifestyle.

5. Harmonise or revitalise
Is there a relationship you would like to heal, a project you would like to enliven, a hobby you would like to renew, a wardrobe you would like to modernise, or a health habit you would like to reclaim? Do you have an aspect of your life that you would like to rejuvenate? Consider today a great day to begin or renew.

Rejuvenat*ion* Summary

- Life is a process not a product.
- Invite family and friends to share food. It unites in conversation and connection.
- Try an adventure that you have not done before.
- Listen to your body, mind and soul. What do you need and want?
- Find a wellbeing activity that suits you and your lifestyle.

5 gems to create 'soulitude'

43. Relaxat*ion*

Quotation

Relaxation needs to be a priority because you are a priority in your life. If you are not making yourself a priority, then who will, who can? What do you do for yourself to decompress and recompose? – Raelene Dal Santo

Notation

Relaxation and its forms, are as diverse as individuals. It could mean the art of balance, a calming effect on the mind, body and soul. It could mean an escape from physical, emotional, psychological, digital or social fatigue. You could find this by solitude or engaged in a relaxing activity either by yourself or with family and friends, away from the causes of such fatigue.

Thrive on Five

1. Create moments

For some, relaxation is energising movement such as the rhythm in walking, running or swimming. Relaxation is finding the stability amongst the instability. For some, it is finding space for contemplation, creativity and inspiration. It is finding your own way to reduce tension of any kind. Find the moments of joy and peace in your life each day. Be grateful for them and create them.

2. Listen to music

Listen to your favourite music whilst relaxing, exercising, working or being at home. Music stimulates neural pathways and can create and spark creativity and memories. It can be relaxing and calming. Music is a powerful healing tool. What is your favourite type of music? Who is your favourite band or singer? What is your favourite song?

3. Be creative

Draw. Paint. Sew. Build. Write. Dance. Sing. Garden. Construct. Design. Play. Listen to music. Laugh out loud. What creative activity do you enjoy, or would you like to explore? Find an activity that allows your creativity to sparkle.

4. Be in nature

Notice nature. Observe the rhythms of nature and the ebb and flow of life. Watch wildlife. Walk. Run. Exercise. Picnic. Play. Observe. Read. Garden. Sail. Paint. Draw. Write. Swim. Let the outside in. Be outside. Mother Nature has many lessons to guide and teach. Take time out in nature for relaxation. Listen. Notice. Observe.

5. Breathe

Be conscious of your breath. Breathe rhythmically and calmly. Slow down. Calm. Close your eyes. Learn to meditate. Lie. Sit. Relax. Breathe. Try yoga, Qi Gong or Tai Chi. Sleep. Rest. Breathe. A suggested book on breathing for wellbeing is, *The Oxygen Advantage*, by Patrick McKeown.

Relaxation Summary

- Relaxation activities are as diverse as humanity.
- What relaxation activity calms your body, mind and soul?
- Allow yourself time to be expressive through creativity.
- Allow yourself time to be in nature.
- Find peace at your special place.

5 nourishing ways to achieve what you need and want

44. Satisfact*ion*

Quotation
Satisfaction lies in the effort, not in the attainment, full effort is full victory.
– Mahatma Gandhi

Notation
Do you feel fulfilled in your life and lifestyle? Are your needs and wants met by yourself or those that share your life? Do you feel contentment, pleasure and happiness in your life? Do you feel satisfied and have joy in your life? Remember a time when you were so proud and pleased you received or achieved something you needed or wanted. How did you fulfil that need, wish, goal or dream? You can achieve and anything is possible.

Thrive on Five
1. Define satisfaction
What brings joy to your life? Are you okay with life how it is? Are you living your ideal life and lifestyle with the people you love? If so, celebrations for you. If not, are you comparing or judging yourself? Are you working towards a goal or a dream? Living your life, following your dreams and life purpose is something that everyone strives to achieve. The access path to these dreams and ambitions is different for everyone. Value difference. When you achieve a goal, do you celebrate or set another? Life is a series of journeys. The process or the journey may bring contentment and satisfaction, not just the end goal.

2. Live your dreams
For some there is the life you live and the life inside you that wants to be lived. Is the life you are living ideal? What would you like to be, do and have? If there were no limitations and fear did not stop you, what would you do? Answer honestly, without judgement, without 'oh but', without the 'what ifs?' What would you like to do? Be that? What are you waiting for? Stop putting it off. Have that one conversation or take that one action that may change your life. Is it overwhelming? Yes. Is it overwhelming not to? Yes. So, what are you waiting for? Make someday, one day, today! Create it. Plan it. Love it.

3. Needs vs wants
Are your needs and wants fulfilled or are you comparing your life and lifestyle with that of others and the consumer society that abounds? What are your needs? Needs are basic requirements of survival. These include food, water, clean air, feeling safe, clothes for protection and shelter. Wants are what

you would like, either real for you or perceived because others may have them. Examine if your basic human needs are being met, and some of your wants. What gives you satisfaction? Being grateful for what you have may demonstrate what abundance is already in your life. Enjoy your life.

4. A well-being
The feeling of not having something, being insecure and overwhelmed by this, may cause stress, anxiety, even anger and is not conducive to mental or physical wellness. Reflection of your life in terms of what gives you security yet autonomy, and what brings you passion, is a place to begin. What gives you a sense of happiness, fulfilment, pleasure and enjoyment in your life? Follow the pursuits that brings your heart fullness. Seek out what you need.

5. Ask for help
Being vulnerable, fearing rejection, feeling overwhelmed, or fear of being a burden, are all reasons that could stop you asking for help. It is counterproductive because to achieve, everyone needs help. We are all interconnected. Sharing you don't know how to do something, asking for guidance, questioning and being willing to listen and learn, brings you closer to satisfaction. Everyone needs help with something.

Satisfact*ion* Summary
- Are your basic needs of survival being met?
- Define your version of satisfaction.
- Be grateful for what already exists in your life.

LIVE WITH LOVE

- Are you being responsible for your own wellbeing?
- What are you waiting for?

5 reminders of learning life lessons in every moment

45. Self-realisation

Quotation
Happiness is not found outside, seek it from within. – Buddha

Notation
A question asked by millions daily is 'Who am I?' It is a source of awareness, to attaining self-realisation. For this notation, I am not qualified and could not give justice to the various theories, forms and ways of self-realisation, other than to say that the ability to reason, allows humans to look at existential deliberation and contemplation. You may like to further research self-realisation, regarding spirituality, psychology, and philosophy; both Western understanding and Eastern understanding (such as Hinduism, Buddhism and Sikhism).

Thrive on Five

1. No manual

Life has no manual but many lessons. The lessons have no schedule and some lessons take time to figure out. Life is a continuum of lessons from the moment you are born until the moment you die. At all times, you are making choices. It would be handy to have a crystal ball with a warning of events but learning lessons from where you have been and where you will go, are all part of the journey.

2. Change perspective

Dr Wayne Dyer said, 'Change the way you look at things and the things you look at change.' Given a different perspective of something, what would you choose to change in your life? If you had no extraneous variables, nor limits restricting your choice, what would you choose to be, do and have?

3. Your gifts and talents

Be present to what makes you truly happy. Are you being true to you? Where and how do you allow your expression of self-realisation to be seen, heard and felt in the world? What gifts and talents are unknown or underutilised, that if allowed to shine would bring joy to your soul? Realising this, is a step closer to sharing your gifts, talents and potential with the world. Allow them to be shared. What is something you have always wanted to learn or share with the world?

4. Love lists

Sit in quiet contemplation in a calming space and place, perhaps with lights low and relaxing music. List the things you love, including people, places, nature and things. Next, write a list of your strengths or character traits, and with each word write an occupation that you know may need this trait. Do not judge your ideas, just write. Give yourself ten minutes to write anything that comes to mind, even if it does not seem clear. You are not the judge, just the audience. Did your list reveal any insights?

5. Self-realisation practices
Some practices allow you to reach a new state of awareness, where you can find inner peace, freedom from fears, spiritual fulfilment, and create stable and calm relationships with others. They can help you feel liberated from worldly attachments, cultural and social pressure, or external influences. Yoga is one such practice that can help you let go of things that identify with the ego and identify with your true self.

Self-realisat*ion* Summary
- Life has no manual.
- Life has lessons.
- Lessons have no schedule.
- Share your 'younique' gifts and talents with the world.
- Life is a series of journeys.

5 ways to monitor, maintain or alter your behaviour in each moment

46. Self-regulat*ion*

Quotation
The first and best victory is to conquer self. – Plato

Notation
Monitoring, maintain or altering your behaviour, thoughts, and emotions in accordance with the situation is self-regulation. It is a complex process of observing, identifying, accepting and managing emotions.

Thrive on Five

1. Self or emotional regulation

Self-regulation is an essential life skill that for some it seems inherent, for some it needs to be an explicit, continual, taught and learned skill. At times, you may need to learn, at times practice and apply the acquired skill or knowledge, and at other times, teach others. Instructor led or self-regulated environments vary in accordance with individual, community or organisational needs.

2. Self-regulation techniques

Being responsible for your own thoughts, words and actions is self-regulation. It is without external control or monitoring, but life is as life does and at times, we all need a little help or reminders. Families and schools can be places where a conscious effort is made to teach and learn self-regulation, guided by metacognition, which is thinking about ones' thinking, and being responsible for your behaviours of thought, words and action. This is a broad subject involving many sub-parts. It is like fashion in that it is very personal. What techniques do you use for self-regulation?

3. Who is your reminder?

Sometimes we can self-regulate, sometimes we all need reminders from family, friends, pets, or nature to remind us that we are always cared for and as my favourite saying reminds, 'The universe always provides.' 'I am okay, and everything is okay.' is another. My Mum is the Quotation Queen and always seems to know the right thing to say to someone in each situation. Her manner is calm, her words are calming. She personifies positivity, acceptance, forgiveness and love. Who in your life is a reminder for you that you are okay, and everything is okay?

4. What is your go to self-regulation tool?
Do you complete self-set tasks? Do you plan? Do you have tools that remind you of events? Do you seek information to help investigate or solve a problem? Do you have tricks that help you remember things? Can you study, work or live with noise and distractions, or do you like calm and quiet? Do you learn by listening, speaking, observing, being involved, or a combination of these? Do you need visual reminders, calming others or a calm place to help you self-regulate? You will choose tools to help you self-regulate. As important, is remembering others may have their own self-regulation tools too.

5. Power is always in the present moment
As a teacher, questioning is a powerful and insightful technique. Asking divergent questions, gives an insight into both teaching and learning, giving an opportunity to self-analyse, problem solve, gauge comprehension and actively engage in teaching and learning. Questioning allows for you to check how your intended message landed, or was it received and perceived in a diametrically opposed way? Is there another way of expressing, teaching or learning? Being adaptable to the other person and the situation is a valuable skill. It is not changing the essence of you but responding to the present situation and where the other person is at. What technique do you or could you choose, to help you be calm and centred, to be present, right here and right now?

Self-regulat*ion* Summary

- Self-regulation is an essential life skill.
- Self-regulation sometimes requires external reminders and influence. Loved ones can be reminders of your reflection in the world.
- Cognitive flexibility, adaptability and creativity are valued skills in relationships and in the workplace.
- Be responsible for your thoughts, words and actions. What are your top three techniques to calm and self-regulate?
- Breathe. Just breathe. A life essential word and action.

5 ways to allow yourself to feel it to heal it

47. Sensat*ion*

Quotation
The great art of life is sensation, to feel that we exist, even in pain. – Lord Byron

Notation
A sensation can be in physical form or from an impression. It can be an awareness in consciousness or something that causes interest. Sometimes it can feel joyous and at other times, painful.

Thrive on Five

1. Comfort

When someone is upset, your natural reaction is to comfort them and at some level wanting to take away their pain. Sometimes the depth of sensation can seem overwhelming and dark. Sometimes the 'feel it to heal it' principle applies and with time and assistance either personal or professional, healing happens. Like all things, healing is a process not a product. Each day is a new beginning. Everyone at times, needs support. You need to honour your own journey and that of another. There are always lessons to learn. Even if each of us have a similar lesson, the situation and circumstances differ. Choosing compassion and self-compassion are gifts both for the giver and receiver.

2. Have a good laugh

Laughter is contagious. If we mimic the characteristics of the people we are with, and consciously and subconsciously pick up on their behaviours and mannerisms then laughter is a great contagion. Josh Billings sums it up, 'Laughter is the sensation of feeling good all over and showing it principally in one place.' When was the last time you had a great big belly laugh? Being around happy, positive people is contagious too and great for the soul.

3. The sensation of nature

Have you ever looked at the stars? Have you ever sat staring at the ocean or floated in it? Have you been alone on a mountain top? Have you ever walked in the undergrowth of a forest? Have you ever noticed and felt the sensation that you are part of a larger picture? Have you noticed the beauty of nature? Notice how nature has the healing power of removing time and holding any human concerns at bay so you can just be in the sensation of now? Be you. Be in nature. Be in the now.

4. Time out. Time alone.
No signal. No devices. No one. Just you. Find space and time so you can be with your inner voice and listen to your inner wisdom. Create this however you can. Find your inner peace and strength. Seek time out. Ask for time out. Choose you. Go somewhere for, and be someone, to you. Read. Relax. Coffee at a café. Walk. Run. Meditate. Take a moment to recharge and do what works for you.

5. Sensation itself
Everyone has something that gives them pleasure and joy. Something that allows you to not think about thinking. Something that provides escape. Something in the moment that is a sanctuary. Something that allows you to completely lose yourself yet be in peaceful control. Something that is soul-hugging. It could be a person, words, music, acts of service, physical contact, gifts, or quality time spent with near and dear. Notice loveliness.

Sensat*ion* Summary

- Laugh. Laugh. Laugh.
- Be with positive, uplifting souls.
- Be in nature. Notice Mother nature's beauty.
- Create time out just for you, for 'soulitude.'
- What sensation gives you a soul hug?

5 guiding ideas on the sameness and newness of habits and customs

48. Tradit*ion*

Quotation
A tradition without intelligence is not worth having. – T. S. Elliot

Notation
Traditions can guide, teach and lessons can be learned. Traditions can become habit and then after time, people become accustomed to things a certain way, sometimes, even when they become unworkable and are unjust.

Thrive on Five

1. Being respectful of traditions

Traversing the globe and conversing with humans and learning to navigate your own humanity and that of others, is a precious gift to yourself and to the world. You will have your opinions, some the same as another, some incongruent. So, whilst you may like or have certain traditions, not everyone appreciates, nor may respect it. Being respectful, even without understanding, allows for the acceptance of someone, some culture, or some country's tradition. Diplomacy is not always easy but is necessary. Perhaps some keys to diplomacy are information rather than ignorance and learning rather than lecturing. Your voice is a powerful tool for standing up for a perceived right, against a perceived wrong. Someone else may agree or disagree. That's life.

2. Be flexible in your thinking

Be flexible in your thinking to know that sometimes you will cling to tradition because of fear of newness or for the joy it serves. Either way the changing to, or releasing of a tradition is personal, it is national, and it is global. Letting go of that which doesn't serve and letting in that which now serves is a skill. Not everyone will see it from your viewpoint. Some people cling to traditions long after it has served its purpose. Personal, generational, cultural or political traditions may have a purpose for a reason or a time. What traditions do you have? What traditions could you let go of?

3. Lessons of tradition

Be mindful of when the lesson is learned, and the tradition no longer serves that which it once supported. These could include personal, familial, cultural, national or global traditions. Are there any traditions in your world that are outdated and served their purpose? Similarly, are there any traditions you could create in your world, or the world, that bring happiness, new lessons and joy to yourself and others?

4. Food traditions

Food connects us in many ways: to our body, our mind, our families, our communities, to the land, and to the traditions of culture. This tradition of food uniting is global. Over time and over lands, these traditions change with the transient nature of people, and the availability or non-availability of ingredients. What food does, is unite people. Food brings people together, in shared conversation and shared memories. Sharing a meal is my favourite tradition and is why I love baking and studied patisserie. Since childhood, I observed how food made by family members united us in conversation and celebration. Do you remember a time food united you, your family and friends for special times? How could you unite your loved ones for congratulation and celebration, to share good times, good food and good company?

5. The heart of traditions

Traditions can build human bridges, yet some can destroy them. At the heart of all traditions is the heart, and if not, then what is? Is it a tradition of compassion or condemnation? Some traditions may seem to stay the same and other traditions seem to be constantly changing. Some of the *'ion'* words in this book are part of the tradition of our daily lives. These include compassion, conversation, expression, celebration, information, as well as empathy, forgiveness, kindness and the overarching one, love. What are your traditions? Do they have a positive or negative affect on yourself or on someone else?

Trad*it*ion Summary

- Traditions can guide and teach.
- Traditions may need to be released.
- Traditions could be commenced.
- Be respectful of traditions although you may not understand.
- Diplomacy is not always easy, but necessary.

5 reminders of the journey not destination of life

49. Transformat*ion*

Quotation
Transformation is a journey without destination. – T. S. Elliot

Notation
How and what do you want to change in your life? Awareness is the key, action is the door and transformation, is the possibility that awaits you. Transformation is a process and like life, a journey. From where, can you source inspiration and use imagination to create newness of interpretation. Be it art, poetry, stories or nature. What is something that makes your soul sing? Live the life inside, that is yearning to shine into the world. Do that thing and be the person that you would like to be. Make someday, one day, today!

Thrive on Five

1. Go within
Transformation requires change. Although change is a constancy in life, choosing to change is transformation. It is not an easy path to travel, yet a rewarding one. If you want to change something, first you need to identify it. It may take time, effort, strength and courage to change. When seeking transformation, ask yourself, 'Does this add to my life?' If yes, great, if not, perhaps a time to let go, reset and renew.

2. Self-transformation
Most people fear change. When you choose to change, some may like you as you are, and some may welcome the transforming process. Fear may come from the unknown in terms of behaviour and expectations. Change is not easy. Change within involves growth. Growth is a process, as you choose to transform something about who you know yourself to be. Each day is a new day for transformation. Be kind to yourself, and others adapting around you.

3. Release old thoughts and patterns
What have you held onto as patterns of thoughts and behaviours that you thought were truths, or you just do them because you thought you had to? What no longer serves you? What is something that if removed, would make way for newness to enter your life? Be it thoughts, things, people or places. Only you will know, and you will know when to let go. Ask for help where needed, both emotionally and for the physical removal of things.

4. Invisible change

No one really knows what happens behind the eyes of someone else. Changes occur within each person all the time. Some transformations of appearance or behaviours can be visible, other transformations invisible, but the effects can be seen or felt. If you notice someone's behaviour is impacting their wellbeing offer help within your capabilities, and if required, encourage medical or health care assistance. Transformations can be joyous. Have you ever had a moment when you felt an emotional 'weight' lifted from your shoulders? A friend described it as, 'The invisible backpack of rocks has been lifted off by back.' I could hear the joy and relief in her voice. This will occur for 'younique' you.

5. Live with Love
Discover what makes your heart sing and find ways to create the life you want. Ask for help where needed and allow others to contribute. This may in turn allow their heart to sing. Harness the magic of the practical activities in this book to transform and live a life you love.

Transformat*ion* Summary
- Transformation is a process.
- Discover what makes your soul sing.
- Transformation requires change.
- Change is a constancy of life and requires energy, courage and commitment.
- Release what no longer adds to your life.

5 ideas to homestay or getaway

50. Vacat*ion*

Quotation
A vacation is what you take when you can no longer take what you've been taking. – Earl Wilson

Notation
Enjoy the hospitality of others, or the retreat to self; to relax, rest and rejuvenate your body, mind and soul. What calls you? Home, mountains, beach, country or remote areas? Listen to your inner voice and choose.

Thrive on Five

1. Plan a holiday

Whether you need to recharge or charge about, plan a holiday. Get brochures. Search the internet. Visit a travel agent. Read an article, blog, newspaper article, magazine or ask family and friends for inspiration. Are you needing a staycation at home, or a state, national or international vacation? Is there somewhere you have always wanted to visit? Be it hidden holiday gems, gastronomic getaways, cultural experiences, physical pursuits, river meanders, ocean cruises, desert wanderings or escape destinations. Country, city, coastal or remote retreats all await you. Plan. Create. Enjoy.

2. Emotional and social vacation benefits

Planning a holiday has a significant emotional impact. When you plan for something you live into that joyous future for yourself and others. Be involved. Discover where and what everyone would like to do. Do what you love. Rejuvenate. Fly. Cruise. Drive. Camp. Trek. Walk. Run. Safari. Explore. Swim. Cycle. Climb. Wander. Learn. Read. What do you need and want from a vacation?

3. Visualise or dream of a holiday

Planning or taking a vacation may not be physically, financially or logistically possible at present. Perhaps now, for whatever reason, you are unable to take a holiday. Create a digital or physical vision board using picture from magazines, newspapers and travel brochures of places you would like to visit. Put this in a visible place so that you can feel the excitement. Enjoy the anticipation.

4. Create a travel account

Nominate an amount you could enter each week. Only use for your well-deserved holiday. A friend saved every five dollar note received and put it in a holiday account. You will be surprised that when you see, receive or transfer five dollars, it will become precious, and soon this small note adds up to a large amount.

5. Budget holidays

Travel to visit a family member or friend. Check regulatory requirements, but consider a house sit or house swap. Plan and take advantage of discounts, or alternatively search websites that offer last minute deals. Go for a drive or a weekend getaway. Remember being physically away can help you to rejuvenate by being emotionally away from familiar daily distractions.

Vacat*ion* Summary

- What place calls you for a vacation? Do you have a favourite holiday destination?
- Is there somewhere you have always wanted to visit?
- Taking time away and digital time out is beneficial to wellbeing.
- A vacation could be from what you do every day, not necessarily to travel away.
- Find moments in your life to be, not just do and have.

5 observances for every breath you take

51. Ventilat*ion*

Quotation
I wake up every day and I think, 'I'm breathing! It's a good day.' – Eve Ensler

Notation
Wherever and whoever you are, good ventilation is essential as it provides oxygen for life. The invisible life force. Breathing is involuntary and vital to sustain life. As mentioned, *The Oxygen Advantage*, by Patrick McKeown shares, how the way you breathe affects your health and fitness.

Thrive on Five

1. Allow air in and out
Breathe. Breathe. Breathe. The breath is vital. Learn to breathe correctly. Learn how to breathe to calm. The exchange of air between the lungs and the surrounding environment or the ambient air is an essential life ingredient. Emotional regulation is a skill that seems innate in some and a continual lesson for others. Find an activity that fits you and your lifestyle. You may like to try Yoga, meditation, Tai Chi or Qi Gong all of which use breath control with a combination of movements. What is something that provides calm for you?

2. Just breathe
The breath of life is essential. Use it as a means of increasing awareness and for calming the nervous system. This simple technique can calm you almost anywhere, at any time. Using the nose only, inhale for a count of four breaths, hold for a count of four and exhale slowly for a count of four. It may distract you from racing thoughts and increase focus.

3. Open the window
Change the air. Allow the ventilation in the room to change so that there is movement of and access to fresh air. Allow fresh air to continuously flow through your dwelling providing newness. Who or what do you need or want to enter your life, that would allow for 'a breath of fresh air?' If your premises are air conditioned, take a fresh air break from time to time.

4. Venting
Venting what frustrates or holds you back, allows for the releasing and in some cases healing, of emotions and feelings.

This could be done personally or in a professional situation with a medical or health care provider. What or who do you need to let go of, release and forgive? Calm breathing helps to create calm.

5. Mind over matter
Often said, often heard, seldom practiced. However, some know it is possible to use the power of voluntary over involuntary. A bit like choosing the possible over what is perceived not to be possible. Like choosing courage in the face of adversity, and as Susan Jeffers book title suggests, *Feel the fear and do it anyway*. Adventurer, presenter and businessman, Todd Sampson (see website), shared in a seminar a couple of years ago, that by using the power of breath and the mind, he can harness the fear and with courage achieve his goals.

Ventilat*ion* Summary
- Oxygen is vital for life.
- Learn to breathe correctly.
- Change the air, both physically and emotionally for optimum health.
- What do you need to vent to release from your life?
- Using your breath and the power of your mind, harness fear and achieve your dreams and goals.

5 lifestyle ideas for your study, job or career

52. Voca*tion*

Quotation
It is not more vacation we need - it is more vocation. – Eleanor Roosevelt

Notation
People often ask, 'What do you do?' Generally, they are referring to your employment, career or occupation. You may know your life work, calling, mission or purpose. For others, their life work may not be clear. Who do you need to be, so you can do and then have what you want for your life? It's okay to know, and yet not know. Wherever you are along the continuum of knowing and not knowing, try to live with love and find ways to access what you want for yourself and those you love. It is your life, live it by choosing to love yourself, to be with those that you love, and love you. Be in work and play that makes your heart and soul sing, dance and play. Have fun. You dedicate a lot of time at work, so love who you are and what you do.

Thrive on Five

1. Be courageous
You choose the direction of your life. What have you always wanted to do or be, but self-doubt, guilt or fear has held you back? What have you been afraid of and still went ahead and did something, achieved something, conquered something? Having the courage to overcome fear by stepping towards it, rather than away, makes you stronger than you know yourself to be. It is not what you are doing that makes what you do seem courageous, it is who you are being as you are doing this activity.

2. Today is your day
If today was your only day, what would you do? It is rare that someone thinks about it until a pivotal moment in their life. What if you didn't wait until you suffered loss, grief, illness or injury? Everyone has disappointments, and I thought the words of Dr Seuss from *Oh, the places you'll go*, could be a reminder to you, 'You're off to great places! Today is your day! Your mountain is waiting, so……get on your way!' Be kind to yourself and be kind to others. Everyone is on their journey, in this collective journey of life. Make yours your vocation to enjoy.

3. It is up to me
Only you know your goals, dreams and hearts desires. Only you can allow yourself to live the life you love. Only you know what it is you really need or want. The lesson to learn is that you do not need to do it all by yourself. It is your dream, but allow others to help you achieve it. Enrolling others in your heart's desires may offer possibilities, opportunities and circumstances

that you may not have known could exist. William H Johnson's words may help, 'If it is to be, it is up to me.' Dream it. Share it. Create it. Enjoy it.

4. Oust obstacles
These could be real or perceived. These could be thoughts, words, words of others, beliefs, or influences. Whatever they are, remember your goal or your dream. Henty Ford said, 'Obstacles are those frightful things you see when you take your eyes off your goal.' Be resolute. Be fulfilled. Create that someday, one day, today! *Live with Love* for your dreams. Ask five trusted family or friends to share with you their observations of three of your strengths and three of your perceived weaknesses. Listen without defence. Learn from how you show up in the world to them. They may give you insightful information that you may not know about you. Take note of your talents and develop them. Perceived weaknesses may reduce when you build on strengths and talents.

5. Learn about your options
Read the newspapers and online job agencies for the variety of local, national or international jobs. Does anything ask for the skills, experiences and knowledge that you already have? Discover how your skills could be utilised in other professions and again I recommend, *What colour is your parachute?* by Richard N Bolles. Does a vocation or profession require skills that you would be willing to learn? Are you interested in creating your own business? Listen to your inner guidance.

Voc*ation* Summary
- Choose the direction of your life.

- Who you are being in every moment counts.
- Today is your day.
- Determine your dream and be determined.
- Value your knowledge, skills and experience. Life is a continual lesson of learning.

5. LIFE IS LOVE. LOVE IS LIFE

A state of change

We are all *'ion,'* in a constant state of change. The flow is a positive and negative state, ever changing. Energy is required for physical and mental activity and the changes in energy can affect wellbeing. Other words you may have heard to describe energy regarding a person are vitality, passion, vibrancy, spiritedness and my favourite, sparkle.

Be kind to yourself. Everyday your body is different. Your energy is different. Be with that. Only do what feels right for you in the moment. Sometimes just be, with nowhere to go, nothing to do and no one to be, except someone to yourself in the moment. Allow your mind to be still. Your heartbeat, calm. Your soul, soothed. Be grateful for this moment.

Your relationship with you

The person that you have the longest relationship in life with is you. You. Yes You. Live your life in accordance with your values and what is important to you. Live from self and live in unity from community, whatever that is for you. To connect to yourself and other human beings is the essence of what life is. To serve yourself with love, give love and be loved are important human needs. You are love. To love yourself is the greatest gift you can afford yourself.

With this, love is my favourite word and possibly with no surprise, my favourite song is *All You Need Is Love*, by the Beatles. We all have moral compasses by which we live our lives, and this determines our actions in the world. Mine, yours and someone else's will be different and again this is determined by all factors mentioned that make you an individual. It is refreshing and affirming that in the journey of life you meet like-minded individuals, and this is when your vibe attracts your tribe. We all meet people at all stages of life. People who 'get you,' love you and nurture you. Be grateful when others allow you to contribute to their life. Be grateful when others contribute to your life.

This is the essence and message of this book:
Let the love in your heart shine into your world and let the love of the world shine in your heart. - Raelene Dal Santo

Protect your energy

Forgiveness is the freeing positive gift that lifts the negative bonds of energy attachment. Self-nourishment, self-nurturing and self-love are selfless gifts, not selfish. Protect your energy.

Be well and live well: from a wellbeing perspective, manage and maintain your energy and be led by your inner guidance.

There are medical professionals, wellness courses, health and mindset coaches, energy healers, allied health services and natural therapists you could research, when dealing with difficult situations and people. Asking for help is a gift, to you and to the person you are asking. In this way, they can then contribute to your life and as the saying goes, in giving, you receive.

Your time to journey

Sometimes things in life may seem overwhelming, but just start where you are, keep going and be in aligned action.

Now, it is time for your journey. What next serves you, to *'ion'* your life, right here, right now, so that you can be the best version of you and *Live with Love*?

Everyone is different. What gifts, talents and ideas are yearning inside you, needing and wanting to be brought into the world?

Lao Tzu said, 'The journey of a thousand miles begins with one step.' The journey of your life begins with one step too. What is your next step? I wish you wellness, happiness, kindness, calmness and success. Love, create and enjoy your life.

Whatever you choose to be, do and have; remember to *'ion'* your life and *Live with Love*.

Love Raelene

REFERENCES AND SUGGESTED READINGS

Andersson, Benny; Ulvaeus, Bjorn and Andersson, Stig
Dancing Queen. Song
Glen Studio (1976)

Bolles, Richard N
What Colour Is Your Parachute?
Ten Speed Press (2018)

Bolton, Robert
People Skills: How to Assert Yourself, Listen to Others and Resolve Conflicts
Simon and Schuster NY USA (1979)

Coelho, Paolo
The Alchemist
Harper Collins NY USA (1988)

Day, Deborah
Be Happy Now: Become the Active Director of Your Life
Xlibris Group (2015)

Fox, Mem
Whoever You Are
HMH Books for young readers (2006)

Frank, Anne
The Diary of a Young Girl
Contact Publishing (1952)

Hamilton, Dr David R
The Five Side Effects of Kindness
Hay House UK (2017)

Hay, Louise
The Power is Within You
Hay House Inc (1991)

Jeffers, Susan
Feel the Fear and Do It Anyway
Balantine Books (1998)

Kelly, Paul and Carmody, Kev
From Little Things, Big Things Grow, Song
Australia (1993)

Kondo, Marie
The Life Changing Magic of Tidying Up: The Japanese Art of Decluttering and Organising
Sunmark Publishing (2017)

Lennon, John and McCartney, Paul
All You Need Is Love
United Kingdom (1967)

McKeown, Patrick
The Oxygen Advantage
Little Brown Book Group London UK (2015)

Oliver, Jamie
www.jamieoliver.com

Maslow, Abraham
A Theory of Human Motivation
Psychology Review (1943)

Maslow, Abraham
Motivation and Personality
Harper NY USA (1954)

Ryan Hyde, Catherine
Pay It Forward
Simon and Schuster NY USA (1999)

Sampson, Todd
www.toddsampson.au

Shiparo-Lou, Rosemary
The Mentor Within
Michael Hanrahan Publishing (2016)

Suess, Dr
Oh the Places You'll Go
Random House (1990)

Terry, Sebastian
www.100things.com

van Tulleken, Dr Chris and Rippon, Angela
How to Stay Young in Body and Mind
BBC Documentary (2017)

Walsh, Peter
Let It Go: Downsizing Your Way to A Richer, Happier Life
Rodale Books (2017)

INDEX

Read the following *'ion'* words and choose any that interest or appeal to you.

1. Accommodation p26
2. Action p29
3. Affection p33
4. Affiliation p36
5. Appreciation p39
6. Beautification p43
7. Celebration p46
8. Cognition p49
9. Collection p52
10. Communication p55
11. Companion p59
12. Compassion p62
13. Congratulation p65
14. Connection p68
15. Consumption p71
16. Cooperation p75
17. Creation p79
18. Detoxification p82
19. Direction p85
20. Education p89
21. Energisation p92
22. Expression p96
23. Fashion p99
24. Generation p102
25. Hydration p106

26. Impression p109
27. Information p112
28. Innovation p116
29. Inspiration p120
30. Location p124
31. Meditation p127
32. Motion p130
33. Motivation p134
34. Nutrition p138
35. Observation p142
36. Opinion p146
37. Organisation p150
38. Passion p154
39. Preparation p157
40. Protection p160
41. Reflection p164
42. Rejuvenation p168
43. Relaxation p171
44. Satisfaction p174
45. Self-realisation p178
46. Self-regulation p181
47. Sensation p185
48. Tradition p188
49. Transformation p192
50. Vacation p195
51. Ventilation p198
52. Vocation p201

ABOUT THE AUTHOR

Raelene Dal Santo is the Founder of *Wellbeing Ways Australia* which provides information and inspiration for you to transform your wellbeing, connect with what matters and thrive in your world.

As an accomplished Australian educator, Raelene guides individuals to connect with their family, friends and community, and most importantly to themselves.

In *LIVE WITH LOVE: Self Care Guide Highlighting 52 'ion' Wellbeing Words,* Raelene shares her passions, qualifications and experience in writing, hospitality/patisserie and as a registered teacher and massage therapist.

Guiding like a lighthouse, her words are for you to 'Let the love in your heart shine in your world and let the love of the world shine in your heart.'

Raelene loves to bake and has a reputation as a 'Friand Friend,' sharing these award winning delicious golden morsels. Whilst not fat free, it is gluten free and can be eaten, guilt free!

Love, create and enjoy your life. *Live with Love* and *'ion'* your life.

Follow Raelene at Wellbeing Ways
Instagram @wellbeingways
Facebook @wellbeingways
www.wellbeingways.com.au

LIVE WITH LOVE

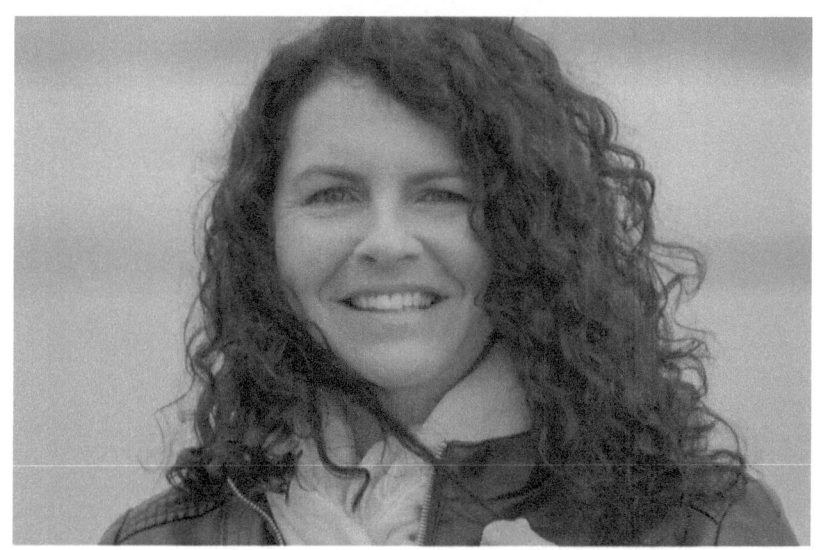

www.ingramcontent.com/pod-product-compliance
Lightning Source LLC
Chambersburg PA
CBHW031414290426
44110CB00011B/382